Physician Heal Thyself

Physician Heal Thyself

By Dr. Hugh Faulkner
with Marian Faulkner

One Peaceful World Press
Becket, Massachusetts

Physician Heal Thyself

Published by One Peaceful World, Becket, Massachusetts, U.S.A.

For further information on mail-order sales, wholesale or retail discounts, distribution, translations, foreign rights, and dramatic and performing rights, please contact the publisher:

One Peaceful World Press
P.O. Box 10
308 Leland Road
Becket, MA 01223
U.S.A.

Telephone (413) 623-2322
Fax (413) 623-8827

Second Printing May 1994

ISBN 0-9628528-6-4
Printed in U.S.A.

Contents

Foreword

As we enter the final decade of the twentieth century, the world is poised at the threshold of a new era. The time is rapidly approaching when the dream of a planetary commonwealth based on health and peace can at last be realized.

However, the road to one peaceful world will not be easy; enormous problems need to be solved before we can enter this new era. Destruction of the natural environment continues day in and day out, while huge nuclear stockpiles still exist even as the Cold War fades into history. The family, the most precious of human institutions, is on the verge of collapse, and in an age of unprecedented prosperity, millions of people don't have enough to eat or a place to live.

At the heart of these global problems is a chronic decline in the health of modern humanity. The modern health crisis is far deeper than problems of inequality in the distribution of medical technology or the astronomical cost of modern medicine, which according to President Bush in his 1992 State of the Union address, reached $800 billion in 1991 and will *double* to $1.6 trillion by the year 2000. The rise of modern degenerative diseases — especially cancer, heart and cardiovascular disorders, mental illness, and more recently, AIDS and immune deficiencies — has occurred even as medical science and technology have continued to develop. In fact, the appearance of these conditions parallels the spread of our modern way of life, including the modern diet, around the world.

When I came to the United States more than forty years ago, cancer affected about one person in seven. At the turn of the century, when agriculture was largely organic and food was still traditional and natural, it affected only one in twenty-five. Now, in the age of high fat, highly refined foods, microwave cooking, irradiated foods, and genetically engineered, chemical agriculture, one out of three people will develop it. Through the 1990s, over a million new cases of cancer can be expected in the United States every year, and the number keeps increasing. If this trend is not reversed, by the year 2000, every other person may develop cancer.

As a result of these statistics, and of the individual suffering caused by cancer, people everywhere are seeking new approaches to prevention. Current research linking cancer to diet and other life-style habits confirms the macrobiotic view that the disease does not strike at random, but results largely from our day to day actions, including, perhaps most importantly, our choice of foods.

Evidence linking the modern diet with cancer continues to mount. In 1977 the United States Senate reviewed the evidence and issued a landmark report entitled, *Dietary Goals for the United States,* in which six of the ten leading causes of death in the United States — including several of the most common cancers —were linked to the modern diet. The Senate Committee suggested that dietary change — especially increasing the intake of complex carbohydrates, such as whole cereal grains, beans, and fresh local vegetables, and reducing consumption of saturated fat, cholesterol, and refined sugar — could lower the risk of cancer and other chronic diseases. These recommendations parallel the nutritional guidelines of macrobiotics.

Similar conclusions were presented in the National Academy of Sciences' 1982 report, *Diet, Nutrition and Cancer,* and in subsequent reports and dietary guidelines issued by the U.S. Surgeon General, the National Cancer Institute, the American Cancer Society, and other public health agencies in the United States, Western Europe, and throughout the world.

The key to preventing cancer can be found not in the laboratory, but in the kitchen. For over thirty years, my associates and I have presented a traditional approach to food and cooking that fulfills the preventive dietary guidelines of these public health agencies. This approach is known as "macrobiotics," from the ancient Greek word meaning "long or great life." It is based on the use of whole cereal grains, beans and bean products, fresh local vegetables, sea vegetables, and other whole natural foods.

The macrobiotic way of eating, which is low in fat, cholesterol, chemical additives, and high in complex carbohydrates and fiber, has successfully — and enjoyably — been adopted by hundreds of thousands of people in dozens of countries, from Russia to Saudi Arabia, from Thailand to Argentina, and from Ireland to Australia. In North America and Europe, more than 15,000 natural food stores and cooperatives now offer high quality macrobiotic staples to an ever expanding number of people, while a network of over 500 macrobiotic educational centers offers guidance to people in many countries around the world. At the United Nations in New York, an international macrobiotic society has been formed to offer this way of life as a solution to problems of world health and peace.

Today, a worldwide consensus is building that a naturally balanced diet along the lines of macrobiotics could help everyone lower their risk of cancer. As I point out in *The Cancer Prevention Diet*, (St. Martin's Press, 1983; revised, expanded, and updated edition, 1993) and *The Macrobiotic Approach to Cancer* (Avery Publishing Group, 1992), whole grains, the staple in macrobiotic kitchens, contain beneficial fiber which lowers the risk of colon and other digestive cancers. In a study conducted in Japan, miso, a traditional seasoning for soups and other dishes, was shown to reduce the incidence of stomach cancer; other studies have shown that sea vegetables, also a part of the macrobiotic diet, inhibit the development of tumors. Moreover, orange, yellow and green leafy vegetables, such as squash, carrots, and others containing beta-carotene, have also been shown to reduce cancer risk.

Evidence that a macrobiotically balanced diet may not only prevent cancer, but may have a positive influence on the outcome of already existing cancers, is now emerging. In a Tulane University survey of twenty-four patients with pancreatic cancer who began macrobiotics, 54 percent were found to be alive at the end of one year, compared with a national tumor registry rate of 10 percent. The researchers who conducted the study called the results "highly statistically significant." Further studies are, of course, necessary, and the Kushi Foundation in Massachusetts will be happy to cooperate with medical organizations in conducting research into the potential benefits of the macrobiotic way of life.

Over the years, I have met many exceptional cancer patients who began the macrobiotic way of life, overcame the odds, and went on to lead normal, healthy and productive lives. Their stories have been published in books such as *Cancer Free: 30 Who Recovered from Cancer Naturally* (Japan Publications, 1992), as well as in newspaper and magazine articles. Dr. High Faulkner, a former London physician now living in Italy, is an outstanding example of an exceptional patient. Dr. Faulkner was diagnosed with cancer of the pancreas. Being a physician, he was aware that medically there was little hope of recovering from his illness, and that the usual rate of survival after diagnosis of pancreatic cancer is from two to four months.

I first met Dr. Faulkner and his lovely wife, Marian, in 1987, at a seminar I was giving for physicians in France. He had met one of my American associates, Edward Esko, at the Community Health Foundation in London several weeks earlier, and had started to practice macrobiotics. I was impressed by his strong native constitution, his clear understanding, and his dedication and compassion for others. These factors, together with Marian's love and devotion to her husband, made me hopeful about the possibility of Dr. Faulkner's recovery. I explained to the Faulkners that the macrobiotic way of life was not a treatment or a therapy, but a common sense approach to living and eating in harmony with nature. They both understood and together embarked on the adventure of a new way of life, with a very happy outcome.

Dr. Faulkner's story is told with clarity, humor, and passion. It offers hope and inspiration to everyone, and can serve as a bridge between modern medicine and the traditional way of life represented by macrobiotics. It advances the development of a medicine for humanity that can turn our modern world crisis toward an age of global health and peace. The dream of a healthy and fulfilling life belongs to everyone. It is my hope that Dr. Faulkner's book, and others like it, will help people in every part of the globe realize this dream, and bring humanity one step closer to one peaceful world.

Michio Kushi
Brookline, Massachusetts 1992

Introduction

The first part of this book is the story of my attempts to escape from a death sentence, together with the reactions of my wife, Marian, who has played a vital role. We offer no magic cure, no panacea for all the ills of mankind. Under the threat of death, I completely changed my diet and lifestyle and to a great extent, my ways of thinking. Has this caused my cancer to go into remission? I don't know. Is this new lease on life — more energy and more ideas — due to macrobiotics? Again, I can't prove it scientifically. Certainly I cannot guarantee that others with cancer can repeat my experiment. Yet I have learned enough from my own experience and from reading and discussions on macrobiotics and traditional Oriental medicine to realize that Western medicine can learn a great deal from these disciplines.

Because I have been a general practitioner for many years and Marian has been a nurse, we have inevitably looked at macrobiotics on the basis of our professional training and experience. I have not abandoned the orthodox Western medicine I was taught at medical school fifty years ago. The spectacular advances in the diagnosis and treatment of disease have clearly helped many thousands of people throughout the world. Yet the cartesian Newtonian concepts on which Western medical science is based have left many gaps — especially in the field of prevention of disease and the promotion of health. Undoubtedly, Western medicine will continue to demand proof that complementary medicine is effective, a demand that is entirely reasonable. The constructive dialogue developing between orthodox medicine and the alternative scene must be encouraged and extended.

My colleagues in macrobiotics should continue to question everything, including their most cherished beliefs. In this they will find allies among doctors and other health workers, and in the universities and research institutes. Medical scientists are not all blinkered reactionaries waiting to pounce on the unorthodox; we all know only too well that no one has the monopoly on wisdom and truth.

I believe that macrobiotics can help many people suffering from cancer. When patients consult me I tell them the facts as I see them. I advise them to talk to their doctor before embarking on macrobiotics, hoping they will find the open mindedness and encouragement I have had from my doctors at the Whittington Hospital in London. Some patients, faced with the realization that orthodox medicine has little to offer, may feel, as I did, that they have nothing to lose in trying.

In the second part of the book I have tried to describe the macrobiotic movement today as I see it, something of its history, and more important, its potential. In addition to its direct role in the field of health, I believe that it can play an important part in the ecology movement, the preservation of our planet from exploitation and war, and the building of one peaceful world.

Hugh Faulkner
Greve in Chianti
Florence, Italy

Chapter 1
The Story

Told by:
Hugh Faulkner: patient and doctor
Marian Faulkner: wife and nurse

"The doctors tell me that all they have to do now is to find out what the body knows that they don't know and then the stuff will be easy to manage." — From James Thurber's last published letter (July 1961) *Selected Letters of James Thurber*, Penguin 1984.

Hugh: The radiologist seemed rather bored with yet another routine, probably unnecessary, ultrasound scan. Suddenly he stopped and concentrated on one area of my abdomen. He didn't tell me what he had found but got up and left the room. When he came back he asked me to go back and see my doctor immediately. We learned from the doctor that the radiologist had seen a mass in the region of my pancreas, a mass which was almost certainly cancerous. He advised an immediate operation. When Marian asked him what would happen if I didn't have the operation, he said that I would almost certainly obstruct. (In effect, the tumor would grow and eventually block the digestive system and flow of bile. Indeed, he was surprised that I had not obstructed already.)

I knew that I could expect to live only a few months, with or without the operation. Cancer of the pancreas frequently presents with few if any signs or symptoms and is, therefore, only diagnosed late. No one can reach the age of seventy-four without accepting the fact that he or she is not immortal. But a death sentence still comes as a profound shock. In a medical journal, I read about a series of American cases where the average survival time after diagnosis was between two and seven months. Few patients survived longer than a year and very few longer than two years. Less than 6 percent of all cases survived more than five years. Although it seemed unlikely that the tumor would prove to be operable, we decided to take the surgeon's advice and go ahead with the operation because of the threat of obstruction.

The ultrasound investigation was carried out at the Whittington Hospital in North London on January 30, 1987, the day before we had planned to return home to Italy by car. I had had some intestinal problems for some years but previous investigations had revealed no obvious organic cause, and I was clearly a candidate fore the diagnosis of "irritable bowel syndrome," often used by doctors as a convenient label for intestinal complaints they don't understand. I had almost convinced myself that my troubles were psychogenic. Almost, but not entirely, because I was happier than I had ever been and had no obvious reason for stress or anxiety.

I had retired at the age of sixty-four after nearly thirty years in general practice in London. After a fairly straightforward divorce, I had married Marian, a nurse with whom I had worked for twenty years. Just before the property boom in Tuscany I had found, almost by chance, a ruined peasant farmhouse in Chianti at a price I could just afford. It nestles on a mountainside, some two thousand feet above sea level, with breathtaking views of wooded hills and distant mountains. After fifteen years, we still never tire of the continual changing patterns of mist and light and shade.

The ultrasound examination that revealed my cancer was almost an afterthought. A colleague was worried by my loss of weight and, despite the fact that previous tests had revealed no abnormality, persuaded me to consult the gastro-enterological unit at the Whittington Hospital in London. Though routine examination and tests revealed no abnormality, my physician, Dr. Beck, ordered the ultrasound because an observant radiologist had spotted a possible filling defect in my barium enema.

The operation was performed on February 3, 1987. We spent the previous weekend informing our nearest and dearest. We wanted the family and close friends to hear the news, however grim, from us personally. John Cochrane, my surgeon, performed the operation himself. He found a tumor "the size of a cricket ball" in the head of the pancreas. He took a specimen for biopsy which subsequently proved histologically to be an adenocarcinoma, a type of cancer. He decided that it was not practical to attempt to remove the tumor, and performed a double bypass to reduce the risk of future obstruction.

I remember very little of the early days after the operation. Whenever I woke up, Marian seemed to be beside my bed, and her presence was enormously comforting to me. The ward was old and full and short of nurses. It contained both medical and surgical patients, some very ill.

Marian: Looking back, my immediate reactions to the news that Hugh had cancer of the pancreas were rather negative. I was afraid he might even die during the operation or soon after. I prepared myself for the worst, reminded myself of the many wonderful years we had had together, and felt very grateful for them. Then, I wondered if I had taken in all the facts correctly. It is not always easy even for nurses, to understand what specialists say. They probably think we know a lot more than we actually do. When something serious arises, I want to be told the facts slowly, so that I can take them in in my own time. I think this is true for many people; they can't fully grasp the situation. Even if they understand the words, they can't yet accept them emotionally. At first it is all rather a shock and almost exciting, and most of us need time to go over things again and again.

There were questions I would have liked to ask the doctors — such as, "What quality of life can Hugh expect during these last few months?" — but I held back, thinking that it was not the right moment, that I should wait for a time when the doctors were less busy. Also I needed to think out and prepare my questions so as not to waste their valuable time.

The hospital specialists gave us virtually no hope. I accepted the fact that little time was left. It seemed that the only thing to do was to try to make Hugh's last few weeks or months as happy and comfortable as possible. I didn't really want to go on living if he was very ill, in pain or unhappy. I've known people who still want to live even when they are in great pain and misery. I expect they hope that things will improve. I was afraid that this period in Hugh's life could be just horrible.

Hugh: After the operation I lost about ten kilos of weight. Marian tells me that I presented a picture of terminal illness to my visitors from my hospital bed. I was blissfully unaware of this. However, as she says, we began to prepare for my imminent death. While I was still in the hospital, we both agreed on the fundamentals. No concealment was feasible or desirable. All concerned should be told the facts, as we knew them, as soon as possible. Once discharged from the hospital, I should inform myself fully on the prognosis and any possible treatment, though we already knew that orthodox medicine had little to offer.

I had already told Marian that if I had a incapacitating terminal illness, I would prefer to be in a hospital or a hospice where I would be cared for by professionals who had chosen to work with the terminally ill, and who would be generous with analgesics and sedatives. I have always greatly admired the pioneering work of Cicely Saunders in the hospice movement and have known of those who have died in peace and dignity in one of her homes. As a general practitioner, I had always respected the expressed desire of patients to die in their own beds, but had too often seen this throw an enormous burden on the spouse or other relatives or friends. Personally, I would much prefer to maintain my dignity and coherence as long as possible with my family and friends during what would hopefully be long visiting hours, whatever trials and tribulations incontinence and general loss of autonomy might bring. Moreover, Marian and other visitors could bring in a breath of fresh air from outside and not be ground down by sleepless nights in a losing battle.

So we decided to find out about hospices and had excellent reports of Edenhall in Hampstead. After my discharge from the hospital, I telephoned this hospice, explained the situation, and was told that I would be accepted at any time we chose. This gave us some sense of security in unknown territory. At least I had the possibility of dying with some dignity as conveniently as possible. It did not seem at all negative or defeatist at the time. I had heard that Edenhall had some kind of religious basis, but when I told them that I subscribed to no church or religious faith, I was assured that this would make no difference.

Marian: Hugh really felt it would be better for us both if he could be looked after in Edenhall when it came towards the end of his life. I, like most people, wanted to be close to my husband when I thought he needed me most. I wanted to do the necessary nursing or caring, and felt that this was really my role. However, I could fully understand his point of view and would naturally respect his wishes. He would so much prefer to have me visit him looking refreshed, with outside news to discuss and time to sit and be with him. If I could do this and give him encouragement and help during these visits, he would have something to look forward to. We had also heard about domiciliary care for the terminally ill and were prepared to find out more about it later on. Now this all seems so long ago, and we have, at least for the moment, put it at the back of our minds.

While Hugh was still in the hospital recovering from the operation, I worried about his children and grandchildren. Should they see him looking so very ill? What if he's actually dying? Should this be their last memory of him? Is he well enough to decide when he wants to see the family or should I decide for him? We had had such a positive and happy life together that in spite of the natural grief I experienced at the thought of losing him, I was comforted by the thought of having relatives and friends near me. And I had a background of Theosophical teachings which I hoped would enable me to face my life with a certain degree of calm and wisdom. I had so much to be grateful for but I had the constant worry that Hugh was almost certainly bound to suffer.

We had, of course, discussed the possibility of Hugh dying in our remote farmhouse in Italy or in the local understaffed hospital, but it seemed more sensible to be nearer our families in London. We were already known at the Whittington Hospital and Hugh had a place booked at the Edenhall hospice, so if it became necessary we could return to London.

From the beginning, Hugh talked so positively about his imminent death. It appeared to be just another adventure for him. This was helpful to us all, especially to our friends and family with chronic illnesses. They felt that they themselves could discuss their life and their own death more freely.

Hugh: We had spent most of our savings and worked hard in restoring our centuries old cottage in Italy. We had worked part-time in the Italian National Health Service since its creation in 1978, and we had many Italian friends. But if I turned out to be at the bottom of the averages and had only a short time to live, (with metastisis and rapid deterioration), a remote farmhouse in Chianti was clearly not the most sensible place to be, no matter how much we loved it.

Looking back at this period, I was not consciously afraid of the act of dying, though I have a normal dislike of pain and suffering. The greatest threat was loss of autonomy. I had seldom been ill, or taken pills or potions. As a doctor I was privileged, both in my access to information and in the speed with which my diagnosis had been acted upon. I was fortunate, too, in that it never occurred to me to give up, to wallow in self-pity or ask why this had to happen to me. In fact, in this period after the operation, we were kept busy trying to organize our remaining life together as well as we could, and therefore, had little time for introspection.

I had had no faith in a personal deity since my teens. My Christian pacifism did not survive the war in Spain, and I had no doubts on the need to defeat fascism by military means, although as a doctor I was never called upon to be an active combatant. I have, however, immense faith in what George Bernard Shaw called "the life force," and in the ability of nature to create an environment in which all living beings can survive, provided it is not ruthlessly destroyed by man for power and profit.

I believe, too , in the almost unlimited capacity of human beings for growth and change, once supplied with the basic needs of life. The frantic accumulation of wealth and consumer goods, whether by hard work or lucky gambling, has never appealed to me. Often it seems to bring not happiness and contentment but fear and anxiety that you will lose all your gains. Despite the superficial attractions of consumerism and what has come to be known as Thatcherism, it will become increasingly clear that it cannot resolve the basic problems of our society.

I feel no need for personal immortality, whether in an afterlife in heaven or subsequent lives on this earth. I am entirely content that the collection of organic matter which has been Hugh Faulkner should return to the common pool of life — giving constituents, that life should go on through my children and my children's children. This is all the immortality I need. However, this does not mean that I was reconciled to dying before I had expected to. We were living in a beautiful place, our family had grown closer and more supportive because of my illness, and we had many unfulfilled plans for work and enjoyment.

Marian: Then Adam Frankenberg came to see Hugh. The son of close friends, Adam is eight years old and suffers from neurofibromatosis. Hugh is like a grandfather to him, and as both were concerned about death, they talked about it. Adam, his five-year-old sister, Rebecca, and their parents, Ronnie and Pauline, were a great comfort to us.

A friend asked me how I actually felt when we learned that Hugh had cancer of the pancreas and that nothing could be done. I had to say that I was not conscious of feeling very much more than I have described already. From the first moments we were busy trying to re-organize our lives. Perhaps I did not allow myself to give way to despair because I wanted to concentrate on helping Hugh all I could, on being positive about his rehabilitation from the operation and his remaining life.

Hugh: Even before any alternative had emerged, we had agreed that the quality of my remaining life was more important than its duration. Whatever the cancer was up to, I decided to try to recover as far as possible from the operation. Many years ago, I helped the orthopedic specialist, Ian Winchester, start a rehabilitation and resettlement clinic at the Whittington Hospital. A small, but enthusiastic, physiotherapy department cooperated fully, and most of the patients who needed rehabilitation could get it in the hospital or at a nearby day-center, as well as advice on re-employment.

While I was still in the hospital, a young physiotherapist taught me respiratory exercises, but when she learned that I was a doctor, she decided that I didn't need them! However, I asked about post-operative rehabilitation and was firmly told that these days there was no time for such refinements. We had previously bought a book on shiatsu by Yukiko Irwin and tried the techniques recommended on one another for neck and back and found them very helpful. Shiatsu combines therapeutic massage with the principles of acupuncture. By massaging acupressure points, it is said that the flow of electromagnetic energy around the body, known as Ch'i in China, and as Ki in Japan, is enhanced. I found that it relieved pain and tension, and I thought it would be ideal for post-operative recovery. Therefore we decided to try to find someone who would give me a shiatsu massage at home. We discussed the problem with my old friend, Avis Hutt, a retired health visitor tutor who is helping us with our research on old people and whom I have known for more than forty years. She rang the Marsden Hospital, the temple of orthodox cancer treatment, and rather surprisingly, spoke to someone who suggested the Community Health Foundation. We learned later that it is the home of macrobiotics in London.

I duly telephoned the Community Health Foundation, as recommended, and spoke to Hilary Totah, who happened to come into the office at that moment. We discovered later that

Hilary is a well known shiatsu practitioner, with a busy life of classes, seminars, conferences and private patients. She lives in the borough of Camden and agreed to come and give me shiatsu in my brother-in-law's house where I was still in bed, shortly after my discharge from the hospital. The first treatment gave me immediate relief from pain and stiffness, and we booked further sessions at home and then at Hilary's house. As she was preparing to leave on the first occasion, she said, "Of course you do know that shiatsu doesn't relieve cancer?" I said that we had never thought it could. She said, "But have you thought about macrobiotics? If you like I can arrange for you to see someone at the Community Health Foundation who will explain its role in the prevention and possibility of recovering from cancer." I said that I had never heard of macrobiotics, and would rather read about it before I met an enthusiastic practitioner. So Hilary provided me with a couple of books and Marian bought another from a local bookshop.

The macrobiotic books appeared to claim that health was a result of how we live our lives and, in particular, what we eat. A diet of grains, such as brown rice, barley, millet and oats, fresh vegetables, dried beans, and a range of seasonings, condiments and other natural foods, in moderation, are recommended. The books also included information on a range of Japanese foods that were completely new to us. These included miso, shoyu, seaweeds, tofu and umeboshi plums. It was also clear that I would have to give up meat, dairy food and sugar. When I looked at all the macrobiotic books available I noticed that many were written by Michio Kushi, who I later learned has been instrumental in developing macrobiotics in the United States and also comes to Europe once or twice a year on lecture tours.

Here for the first time I read that macrobiotics believed that the body could be taught to reject cancer—in orthodox medical terms, that we could materially increase the slim chance of "spontaneous regression." Lying in bed I read all three books from cover to cover. It seemed that I had nothing to lose by giving the macrobiotic diet and way of life a trial. We discussed this with our families and friends and with my general practitioner,

Don Grant, a very old friend and ex-partner. All agreed that since the tumor was inoperable and no chemotherapy or radiotherapy was known to be effective, orthodox Western medicine offered no hope.

John Horder, another old friend and ex-colleague, thought that it would be useful to have an objective opinion on macrobiotics from someone outside its ranks, so we consulted Dr. Patrick Pietroni, a general practitioner who was the founder and first president of the Holistic Medical Association. He assured us that the macrobiotic movement was completely respectable and sincere, but that he knew of no evidence, other than anecdotal, that the macrobiotic diet and way of life could influence an established cancer such as I had. When Marian asked him if he would try macrobiotics if he was in my position, Dr. Pietroni replied: "Probably not." Despite this rather lukewarm opinion, we decided to go ahead. Macrobiotics appeared to offer the possibility of recovery, however remote. Here Marian's enthusiasm and support were vital. She was far more ready to become a believer than I was. So we went to the Community Health Foundation and ate in their excellent macrobiotic restaurant which is open for lunch and evening meals. We also bought more books at Genesis, the bookshop in the same building, and patronized Clearspring, the macrobiotic food store next door.

Marian: I had no idea then that we could have such an appalling diagnosis followed by the five most exciting and happy years of our lives. One fascinating thing has been Hugh's attitude toward complementary medicine and his readiness to meet new problems and challenges. Before working in our London health center as a nurse, I had taken part in faith healing, sometimes referred to as spiritual healing, with animals and with people. I worked as an assistant to a well known healer. Later, I studied meditation, yoga, spiritualism and Eastern philosophy. Then I became a Theosophist and a vegetarian. So macrobiotics was not as new and strange to me as it was to Hugh, though he had encouraged his patients to try other forms of complementary medicine when he thought it could help or when they suggested it. Hugh accepted macrobiotics as a new challenge right from the start. The family and I were delighted by his energy and determination, and he soon looked so much better that we began to believe a miracle was really happening.

Hugh: On March 5, 1987, a month after my operation, I saw Dr. Beck and Mr. Cochrane again at the Whittington Hospital. We told them of our decision to try the macrobiotic diet and way of life, and they immediately accepted this and agreed that I had nothing to lose. They asked me to continue with the pancreatic enzymes to replace any possible deficiency caused by the damage to the pancreas and to aid digestion. They asked me to come back and see them periodically to check my progress and the adequacy of the diet for normal requirements, though they could hardly have expected my visits to have continued for so long. Subsequently, John Cochrane prescribed the hormone, tamoxifen, which has already been used in breast cancer with some success. Its use in pancreatic cancer is apparently based on the discovery of estrogen receptors in the pancreas, and some uncontrolled studies on the effect of anti-estrogens on patients with pancreatic cancer. A prospective, multicenter double-blind randomized trial is planned by the Department of Surgery in the Haukeland University Hospital in Bergen to study the effect of tamoxifen, compared with a placebo. This study should provide more accurate information on the possible use of tamoxifen in pancreatic cancer. However, I doubt if it has played an important role in my recovery, but who knows?

On Saturday, March 7, we had our first meeting with a macrobiotic counselor. We had made an appointment to see Jon Sandifer at the Community Health Foundation, but he was delayed out of London and arranged for us to see Edward Esko instead. Edward turned out to be a delightful, extroverted American from the Kushi Institute in Boston. He saw us in the evening after he had been running a whole day's workshop, but gave us his full attention. He had absolutely no doubt that I would recover! He gave us our first advice on the macrobiotic diet and way of life, advised us to take cooking lessons, and recommended that we see Michio Kushi while he was still in Europe. So we began private lessons with Caro Smith, who was then one of the cooking teachers at the Community Health Foundation, in her small kitchen in Kentish Town. Caro is young and enthusiastic, loves cooking and teaching macrobiotic cooking, and we soon became friends. We had eight, three-hour sessions during which Caro demonstrated many of the basic procedures in macrobiotic cooking and we were able to take away the end-products for warming up at home. These individual lessons were clearly costly, but as there was no immediate course available and we planned to return to Italy as soon as possible, this arrangement was ideal.

Like most people, I was used to a diet of a little red meat, chicken, plenty of eggs, vegetables, white pasta, brown bread, regular use of sugar, chocolates, sweets and several cups of coffee a day. My initial macrobiotic diet included pressure-cooked brown rice, rice with barley and boiled millet, steamed, boiled or stewed vegetables, beans cooked with vegetables until soft as in a thick casserole or soup: and vegetable soups seasoned with wakame seaweed and miso, a thick salty paste. We also ate other seaweeds, a salty, sour, pickled plum called umeboshi, tofu, whole wheat noodles, and stewed fruit twice a week. There was a wide range of seasonings and condiments. We drank mainly spring water or bancha tea which is brewed from twigs. I was advised not to have any meat, chicken, dairy food, eggs, sugar, alcohol, spices, biscuits, or refined foods. Surprisingly, at the beginning, I was also not to have fish, bread of any kind, or raw fruit.

I didn't find the transition to a macrobiotic diet very difficult. Cooking has been a hobby of mine for the past fifteen years or so, and, from the first, I saw the macrobiotic cuisine as a new and interesting challenge.

We had both decided to follow the macrobiotic diet and way of life as seriously and completely as we could. This decision was clearly influenced by my death sentence. If there was any possibility that macrobiotics could help my body to resist the cancer, I was determined to give it every chance to do so. In the early days I was far from convinced about the effectiveness of macrobiotics; therefore, Marian's determination and willingness to follow macrobiotic advice was enormously important. As she said, her experience with Theosophy and spiritual healing allowed her to accept the teaching and philosophy of macrobiotics far more easily than I could.

Although I didn't miss eating meat very much, I was happy when Michio allowed me to have fish occasionally. Not drinking coffee presented no problem, though most of us drink a lot of coffee in Italy, I have drunk none for the past five years. We tend to have a few beverages during the day and although I like the taste of bancha tea, I sometimes get bored with it and I don't like any of the grain coffees. Although herbal teas on the whole are not advised, most Italian bars serve chamomile tea which is, on rare occasions, acceptable in our diet, and I quite like it with a sliver of lemon and no sugar. I usually drink this when my Italian friends are having an espresso or a cappuccino, though we usually carry bancha or kukicha tea with us wherever we go.

After a lifetime of addiction most often sugar has been more difficult to give up. I most often use a malt sweetener, usually brown rice syrup or barley malt. In the first year, Michio's embargo on baked foods produced some problems. We eat a lot of bread in Italy. I probably eat more wholemeal bread than I should, and we are trying to reduce that. Unfortunately, tomatoes, potatoes, and other members of the nightshade family, which Michio strongly disapproves of, are some of the most common vegetables in Tuscany. Looking back on the early days, Caro Smith's enthusiasm and obvious enjoyment was enormously important, and right from the start avoided any risk of macrobiotics becoming a grim battle with temptation. But probably the most important fact was that I began to feel much better and energetic than I had for years after only two or three weeks on the diet.

Marian: I, too, enjoyed Caro's cooking classes, though cooking is not my favorite occupation. The first thing I learned, which is very important, is the need to chew each mouthful many,

many times. Then I heard about the art of balanced meals. Next I discovered that only vegetables in season should be eaten. I found these sessions most useful as a general introduction to macrobiotics, and in giving me confidence to manage the meals when Hugh wanted a break from the kitchen. Normally, he does all the cooking, with only occasional help from me. Cooking is his hobby and relaxation. I usually do the shopping, cleaning, washing dishes and clothes and most of the gardening. So I shouldn't feel guilty when Hugh takes over the cooking! But I do sometimes.

On the whole I like the diet better than Hugh does. I'm quite happy with moderate natural tastes and mildly salted and unspiced foods. Fresh ginger is very useful and on occasion, certainly adds a lot to the taste of dishes. Hugh is not so keen on under-cooked vegetables and doesn't like seaweed unless its cooked with other things. I love seaweed and could eat it on its own any time. It is fortunate that we both like tofu (soybean curd), and tempeh (fermented soy beans), and we love all pulses, especially lentils. We enjoy whole grains and usually start the day with porridge, adding seaweed in place of salt and varying the grain or using a mixture which can be wheat, barley, rye, buckwheat, millet, oats or quinoa. We eat a good deal of whole rice as this is a standard in the macrobiotic diet and we like vegetable soups with seaweed and mushrooms, often adding miso which is made by fermenting soy beans with sea salt and adding barley, wheat or rice.

Hugh: My son, Tim, a radiologist in Norway, arrived and expressed his concern about me. Trained in orthodox Western medicine, he accepted the official prognosis. Though he agreed with our decision to try macrobiotics, he obviously regarded it as "clutching at straws."

When I look back at my diary for this period I realize how busy we were — meeting old friends who wanted to come to say goodbye, having cooking lessons, finding new friends in macrobiotics and buying books and provisions at the Community Health Foundation.

Clive Jenkins, the joint general secretary of the trade union ASTMS (Association of Scientific Technological and Managerial Staff) — now merged into the MSF — (Managerial, Scientific and Financial Association) visited me on February 24, obviously to say goodby. Clive is a very old friend of mine, and I was part-time medical secretary of ASTMS for some years. When later he heard news of my recovery, he sent me a telegram of congratulations from North Africa!

It is difficult to say now whether I would have meekly accepted the onset of terminal illness without the discovery of macrobiotics. In our decision to follow macrobiotic advice as completely as possible, we were greatly helped by Marian's brother, Peter Weiss, and his wife, Rosemarie. Peter visited me every day while I was in the hospital and, after my discharge, he and Rosemarie insisted that we use their small house in Kentish Town as an operational base. This involved commandeering their kitchen for several hours a day while we experimented with our early attempts at macrobiotic cooking.

In all this activity, the most important single element was the sensation that I was regaining control of my own body and taking personal action which could possibly — however improbably from the point of view of orthodox medicine — help my body to overcome cancer. Recent reports from the new specialty of psychoneuroimmunology appear to confirm the fact that we can overcome the passive acceptance of inevitable doom by offering patients hope, if not of cure, at least of the possibility of improving the quality of their remaining life.

When the National Health Service is fighting for its survival, it seems ungrateful to criticize the hospital where I have had so much support and understanding from my two consultants, Eric Beck and John Cochrane. But surely a progressive gastro-enterology unit should have the services of a physiotherapist who could initiate post-operative rehabilitation, a dietician who could advise the patient, the family and the ward kitchen on diet, and a social worker to listen to special problems and give advice on how to cope at home. It seems that these things are not a priority today, even in centers of advanced technology.

With some difficulty we managed to book an appointment to see Michio Kushi in the south of France, on the way home to Italy. He was giving a conference on macrobiotics in Bergerac, mainly for French doctors. We arrived to find the conference being held in a rather grand country hotel.

Our room looked our directly onto paddocks in which various various imported animals were installed. We were separated from a large bison only by a single electric cable, which however appeared to keep him effectively contained. Here we heard Michio Kushi lecture for the first time. He has great charm and charisma, and discourages any attempts to make him a guru or some kind of saint. Aveline, his wife, gave cooking demonstrations. She is very small and delightful, in her sixties now, but looks far younger than her age. She told us she came from a humble family in Japan. At home she was brought up on the traditional Japanese diet, similar to the diet she teaches today, though the Western way of life has brought many changes in Japan. Both Michio and Aveline have strong Japanese accents and at first we found it difficult to understand what they were saying, but it was a very good introduction to macrobiotics and we learned a lot.

Marian and I met with Michio. Rather to our surprise, we were not alone. With us were two students and Michio's secretary at the time, Donna Cowan, who took notes. I imagine we could have asked to see him on our own, but in the warm supportive atmosphere of macrobiotics it seemed quite natural and acceptable. Michio listened to my brief history--it was exactly two months since my diagnosis. He looked very carefully at my face and eyes, and examined my abdomen. I asked him if macrobiotics could help me become free of cancer. He said, "No, but your body can."

He then gave us a set of dietary instructions, which his assistant recorded as Michio talked about my particular diet in greater detail. Most of this can be found in Michio's book, *The Cancer Prevention Diet*. The diet basically consists of 50 to 60 percent of whole brown rice or other whole grains, well cooked pulses, and fresh lightly cooked vegetables in season (preferably local and organically grown). On this first occasion there were further restrictions — no flour products such as bread, cakes, biscuits or pizza, and no baked foods to begin with; no animal products, no fish, no raw fruit, no salads, no spices, no tea coffee or alcohol. Pamela Haines, the bestselling novelist, who herself follows macrobiotics, humorously refers to this as the "No No" diet, because every time you ask Michio if you can eat or drink something, he says "No." Some of these restrictions were relaxed in later meetings. Michio also stressed the importance of chewing every mouthful very well, of regular exercise, fresh air, pure water, and weekly shiatsu massage.

Marian: I took the diet very seriously and was determined to help Hugh to stick to it as strictly as possible. We did not always agree about it, and tended to fuss, which naturally irritated him. But, generally, Hugh is far more relaxed than I am about the diet — and indeed about most things in life. However, I try to shop wisely, always with the diet in mind, and Hugh enjoys cooking and eating most of the things I buy or grow.

Our guests usually like to sample our foods, but we try to have non-macrobiotic foods available as well as we do not wish to force our diet on others. There is no doubt that at least in the beginning, macrobiotic cooking takes longer and requires more concentration than ordinary cooking. We like to cook with love and eat with gratitude. We try not cook in a hurry but sometimes have to. This happens to everyone, and we have to find short cuts in preparing and cooking our meals.

Hugh: At the Bergerac conference, we were all given a large file containing the Physician's Macrobiotic Studies Program. Fifty-five doctors and other health workers, mainly French, took part in the conference though the language spoken was English.

We met some very interesting people including Dr. Ken Bailey, a World Health Organization expert in traditional medicine, who arrived by helicopter and gave a fascinating account of dietary problems in Africa.

Dr. Tony Haines, medical adviser to the British Foreign office, was there in a personal capacity. The directors of the Kushi Institutes of both France and Holland were also present. Kushi's son Lawrence, a qualified nutritionist, was there with his friend Bob Lerman, who was the director of the Clinical Nutrition Unit at the Boston University Medical Center. We had some most interesting discussions on the diet and the possibilities of organizing clinical trials. Lawrence told me that doctors in the states often refuse patients access to their medical records.

He gave me a book review from the *New England Journal of Medicine,* one of the most progressive of the orthodox medical journals, which I found most interesting. A Harvard professor, Arthur Kleinman, was reviewing a report on Chinese traditional medicine. The author, David Eisenberg, was apparently the first American medical student to visit China "under the auspices of the Committee on Scholarly Communication with the People's Republic of China of the National Academy of Science." I have not read the report but Kleinman's account of Eisenberg's description of the remarkable feats of the masters of "Ki gong" (the manipulations of vital energy) whets the appetite for more. "These powerful adepts either teach patients to concentrate and strengthen their inner Ki in order to improve their health, or send Ki outward from their bodies to move objects, break slabs of rock, light electric bulbs, or provide anesthesia.... The author's enthusiasm and sensitivity are likely to win over even skeptics to the view that these are phenomena worthy of scientific research that may be medically important. We are entitled to ask why orthodox Western medicine relies only on the reports of one lone medical student, however enthusiastic and sensitive he may be.

All in all, we were greatly helped by this meeting and my encounter with Michio, and set off for Italy and our new life in a very positive spirit.

Marian: The diet and way of life seemed to help us both from the start. We felt very stimulated and, after those grim days in London, it seemed like a miracle. Here was Hugh, still quite ill — not just hanging on, but enthusiastically accepting macrobiotics as a new challenge. Our friends and relatives have given us so much understanding and love, and have come especially to help us through difficult times. Italian friends were prepared to come to London to see Hugh when we thought he was dying, and other friends have come to our home in Italy to help us. We were even offered nursing help and the use of a flat in London. Fortunately, we have always been most welcome guests of my two brothers who live in London, and we usually stay with them.

Hugh: In Italy, everyone welcomed us back warmly though it took them some time to realize I was not yet tottering to the grave. It was a great joy to us both to get back to our house, even with a totally neglected garden. We have pure air to breathe and our water from a deep well, which our friendly builders dug for us after we had consulted a local water diviner. We work in the garden, where there is always wood to be cut, weeds and brambles and creepers to be cleared away, and compost to be managed. In addition, we work part-time with our research group in the local health district.

After joining a local sports club, we began using a championship swimming pool near our office during our lunch hour. Most days the pool is pleasantly warm, even in mid-winter which is important to me since I am more affected by the cold now than I was before my illness. Perhaps this is due to the loss of superficial fat. Amidst all the experts training with their fast crawls and butterfly strokes, Marian and I sedately swim the appropriate number of lengths with our slow, dignified, breast stroke. I even swam twenty lengths some four months after my operation but this was unnecessary bravado, and normally I am satisfied with swimming ten lengths while Marian does sixteen. We find this form of exercise, though rather expensive, extremely useful for keeping fit, and strongly recommend it. We also take part in a local authority keep-fit class twice a week in a school gymnasium near our office. For this we pay ten thousand lire a season, rather less than five pounds. All very good rehabilitation.

For the first year after Michio recommended the diet, we kept to it as closely as we could. In the summer of that year, I had two sharp reminders that my body did not welcome departure from the diet. On the same day I was entertained at an old age pensioners' lunch, I was invited to the British Consul's celebration of the Queen's birthday. The pensioners had heard about my diet and prepared a large dish of whole-grain rice and carrots for me and watched while I ate it! I unwisely helped it down with Chianti wine, the first alcohol I had drunk since my operation. Later, at the Queen's birthday garden party, I could see nothing on my macrobiotic diet and stupidly decided to sample the caviar and Aste Spumante. My stomach objected violently and uncontrollably to these insults in the middle of the party, fortunately in the open air. One of my medical colleagues kindly drove me home in my own car. I made an uneventful recovery, slightly wiser!

My older daughter, Lyn, her husband, and three-year-old son, visited us, and we took a week's holiday to stay with them at Lake Trasimeno, near Perugia, where we have a caravan. I went for a swim in the lake which was rather too cold for comfort, although the Germans and Scandinavians and even Marian seemed to enjoy it. The next day I had a sore throat and a cold, perhaps as the result of the swim. I was due to go to a seminar on smoking in Rome and I did not tell Marian that I was not feeling well for fear that she would discourage me from going to Rome. So I stayed two nights with a friend in Rome who tried to provide a suitable diet for me. We went to a restaurant which claimed to provide macrobiotic food but served nothing of the kind. Another highly recommended vegetarian restaurant had become Indian and non-vegetarian overnight. The seminar was badly organized and offered very little new material. By the time I arrived back at the lake by train, I was feeling very ill indeed. Marian says I was gray and shaky and seemed to be semi-conscious and she even considered admiting me to a hospital. However, she drove me home to bed, leaving the family for another few days at the lake. By the next day I had completely recovered. I can only assume that my autoimmune system was unable to cope with the cold swim, an upper respiratory infection and departures from my diet. I resolved then and there to avoid cold water and treat sore throats, and my diet with greater respect.

In June 1987, I met with Ferro Ledvinka, the director of the Kushi Institute in Florence and virtually the founder of macrobiotics in Tuscany, and perhaps in Italy. He lives near Florence with his English wife and family. I reported that I felt extremely fit and full of energy, and that as far as possible I had kept to the diet recommended by Michio Kushi. Marian was worried that I was eating too much fruit, bread and biscuits. I said that as long as I felt well and my weight was constant, the occasional lapses were unlikely to be doing any harm, and that anxiety about them could do more harm than good. Fortunately, Ferro agreed with this, but advised me to continue to follow the main lines of the diet, at least until we saw Michio again. He also recommended weekly shiatsu so we fixed appointments with Gioachino Allasia, a shiatsu practitioner and macrobiotic counselor who trained at the Kushi Institute in America, and who has become a close friend. The shiatsu sessions were definitely helpful, and Marian usually came to watch and learn. Gioachino also gave us many useful tips and advice on the macrobiotic way of life, and told us of his experiences — both in Italy and in the United States.

Marian: We learned that macrobiotics is about the joy of living. We are responsible for our own lives. Exercise in whatever form should be a pleasure and not a grim duty. We were encouraged to sing a happy song every day, to give thanks before eating, and to be grateful for our difficulties. We can learn a great deal from them.

Hugh: We were due to go to London again to see my hospital specialists in July 1987, and decided to attend the international macrobiotic camp at Lenk in Switzerland on our way. The camp was held on a beautiful site with residential, hostel-type accommodations, surrounded by mountains. It was apparently constructed by the Swiss army and normally used for training recruits. We slept in our camper amidst the trees in the car-park, probably illegally, but no one asked us to move. Macrobiotic cooks and volunteer helpers provided excellent meals in a central living room. A program of varying activities was available.

Participants, including many young people, came from several countries. We met a number of people who were firmly convinced that macrobiotics had helped them to overcome a wide range of conditions, including cancer. We saw no one obviously poor at the camp, and no minorities. At six each morning, a group of us gazed at the mountain peaks lit by the early morning sun as Jon Sandifer led us in Do-In exercises. These exercises are described in Michio's book *The Book of Do-In*. I practice them most mornings, missing them only if I have gone to bed too late the night before, or if it's too cold. Though the exercises require effort, they are so helpful and stimulating that when I omit them I feel that the day has not started properly. I advise any one interested to choose the exercises that suit you best, sometimes vary them according to whim or need, and don't become too anxious or obsessional about them.

Marian: Feeling too lazy to do Do-In, I joined Gioachino's group where we learned chants from various countries. I used to think that all chanting was monotonous, but many of these chants were surprisingly tuneful. During the camp, it was wonderful to watch Hugh's steady improvement in health and vitality, and his joy in taking part in so many activities. We joined in cooking classes and other seminars and I went with a group to collect edible wild plants in the mountains. We made several friends and Hugh was very popular, especially with the younger people. We both enjoyed the camp very much and I was reminded of long past Theosophical camps. We also visited a heated pool in a local spa near Lenk. It had jets of hot water hitting you body at various points, which was very relaxing and good rehabilitation.

Hugh: I had a further consultation with Michio Kushi at Lenk. Michio's firm conviction that I was 40 percent improved was enormously encouraging and reassuring to us both. He asked me to see him again in about six months.

Perhaps the sessions that impressed me most at Lenk were Saul Goodman's seminars on positive thinking. He is a young, extroverted American, director of the International School of Shiatsu, who succeeds in encouraging maximum audience participation. In the first session he said, "Don't believe anything I tell you. Question everything. Don't believe anyone." Someone said, "Does this apply to Mr. Kushi, too?" "Yes, of course," said Saul. "I'll tell him," said the questioner. "He knows," came back the answer. Saul began the second session by saying, "I want you all to write down what you want for Christmas, what you really want regardless of cost or feasibility." Soon after, he asked us to write down what we didn't want. This is a standard technique in some humanist psychology systems in which various psychologists and communicators are evolving their perceptions of the world, of themselves, and their clients. This approach fits in well with the positive thinking of Oriental philosophy. We have met others in macrobiotic circles interested in neurolinguistic programming, one of the recent developments mentioned by Saul. However, it was new to me then and came at an appropriate moment. I still have the notes I made. For the things I wanted for Christmas, I wrote:

A word processor
A compact disc player
Complete recovery
To play the blues harp (the jazz harmonica)
To learn wood sculpture
Challenges of all kinds

What I didn't want included:

A recurrence of my cancer
Illness or death of Marian
Loss of autonomy in illness or old age
Antiques, jewelry, fur coats

After the seminar I told Marian of my Christmas wishes. She said, "Well, if that's what you really want, why not? We can use what you call my savings. I'd much rather we use them for things we can both enjoy now than rather wait until you are dead." So in London we bought a word processor and are writing this book on it. We bought Hi-Fi equipment and are very much enjoying the reproduction provided by compact discs. Then, I got Dave Michelson's name from the Musician's Union; he's the only harmonica teacher listed in London. He is a young man living amongst a confusion of harmonicas and other musical instruments in a newish housing estate in Islington, only a mile or so from the Community Health Foundation. He has a bed available for fellow musicians in need. I had expected tips on how to make some of the exciting sounds the great blues harp players of the past achieved. Instead, I was instructed in posture, breathing, listening and keeping rhythm and urged to learn to read music. This was all closer to the teachings of Do-In than my ideas of learning to play the blues. Dave proved to be the grandson of J.B. Priestley and his mother teaches music therapy for mental illness. We got on very well, though it took me some sessions to learn to bend a note, and my repertoire is still limited. Dave accepted my desire to learn to play the blues harp at the age of seventy-five and seemed to find it not at all odd.

Marian: It was an interesting experience for me to join one of Hugh's lessons with Dave. They obviously understood one another and Dave gave frequent examples of techniques in playing the blues harp. This was very beautiful as well as instructive. I really enjoyed the session, and the tea and chat afterwards.

Hugh: In London I also had shiatsu from Rex Lassale, recommended by Jon Sandifer. Rex is a charming Trinidadian who admits to a revolutionary past. He is a qualified osteopath, and his shiatsu technique was quite different from any other that I had experienced. It was much more aggressive and often painful, with a great emphasis on deep breathing. It was very helpful and stimulating. Incidentally, Rex has now fallen in love with Italy and is moving here. He will be an invaluable addition to the ranks of shiatsu teachers in Italy.

We met several old and new friends in London, often entertaining them at the macrobiotic restaurant in Old Street. One old friend, Oliver Gillie, an extremely well-informed and open-minded health correspondent, is now editor of the health section of the *Independent*. He was very interested in my story, and suggested that I write something for the paper; I promised to think about it. Subsequently, he arranged for a journalist, Barbara Griggs, to interview me in Florence. She wrote an excellent article which was published in the *Independent* in July 1989, and then reprinted in the *News of the World*. These articles resulted in several thousand inquiries at the Community Health Foundation in London. These inquiries were due to Oliver's initiative, for which we are deeply grateful. I have subsequently been interviewed by two Italian newspapers and have been approached about appearing on Italian television.

But to continue our story in 1987. August 3 was one of the few days I wrote in my diary. I am not a natural diarist, rushing to share my innermost hopes and fears with a little book, completing each day in orderly fashion. However, for some reason on August 3 I tried to do this. In a spate of activity of various kinds, under the broad umbrella of macrobiotics, we were still attempting anything and everything that might possibly help to defeat the cancer. The report of a tamoxifen study from Sweden in a medical journal gave the average survival rate of controls as two and one-half to three months from the date of diagnosis. Obviously, I got a great kick out of being very much alive six months after my diagnosis. Saul Goodman said, "Did you get cancer to show what a great guy you are?" Rex Lassalle says I intellectualize too much. "Just be yourself. Be Hugh! Don't try to become someone else."

But I am also a doctor, an amateur epidemiologist and an active campaigner for people's health. Are those of us who discover macrobiotics a special self-selected group? This and many other questions need more research and further dialogue between macrobiotics and Western medicine.

On August 9, 1987, we flew from Heathrow to Oslo, to spend two weeks in Laerdal with my son, Tim; my daughter, Jill; and her three children. Tim invited them to come from London during our visit and paid their fares so we could all be together. We were met at Oslo airport by our friends, Dr. Dag Bruusgaard and his wife, Erli, who took us back to their beautiful, modern timber house by the sea. Dag is a general practitioner and lecturer in primary health care in Oslo and ex-president of the European General Practice Research workshop of which I am a member. We rested with them until Tim came to get us in our Volkswagon, which my daughter, Jill had brought from England. Tim arranged for us to have a nurses' bungalow on the hospital grounds, as his house was full of guests as well as Polish workers who were restoring it. This arrangement was ideal as we could cook our macrobiotic food on our own in peace and quiet. We had a very pleasant fortnight there. One of our happy discoveries was that raspberries and red-currants grow wild along the footpaths in this area.

An ultrasound test that I had in Florence showed some shrinking and liquification of the tumor. During this visit, Tim repeated the ultrasound in the well-equipped x-ray department in his small hospital. It showed further shrinking of the tumor and the liquification in the center. According to Michio Kushi, this dissolving process of the tumor is typical of someone who is getting better. However, as far as I know, this process is not generally understood in scientific terms.

We returned through Germany and were glad to be home after a very eventful trip — still less than seven months after my operation. In September we organized a workshop on the loss of autonomy in old people as part of our research project. Bob Gann, the very enterprising librarian who started "Help for Health" in Southampton, came. His expenses were paid by the British Council in Rome. Our good friend Paul Wallace, director of the Helen Hamlyn unit in London for research on old people also took part. The workshop was reasonably successful and well-attended, and I was pleased to find that I could take such events in stride.

Albert Kushlick, another great friend who is a psychiatrist working in mental handicap research, came to see us. He is firmly convinced of the value of positive thinking, affirmation and meditation, and says these have all helped him recover from several attacks of coronary thrombosis. He, too, has had to deal with threats of early death, and I found our discussions immensely helpful and encouraging. Although he has not adopted macrobiotics, much of his thinking about illness and handicap is very close to macrobiotic teaching and practice. He believes that people should be responsible for their own health and play an active part in their recovery.

At the end of March 1988, we set off again in our camper for England, along with our good friend Gigi Passerini, a general practitioner in Sondrio, North Italy. Gigi, an excellent driver, drove most of the way since he enjoys driving. We carried out a tightly packed study tour involving long sessions with general practitioners in Birmingham, South Wales and Devon. Out of this will come, we hope, a book for general practitioners in Italy, *A New Type of Doctor*, mainly based on the book with the same title already published in Britain by Julian Tudor Hart, a General Practitioner in Wales who is another long-time friend. Once again I was pleased to find that I could concentrate for long hours without any ill effects. One of our General Practitioner hosts was so impressed that he recently asked advice about his partner's wife who has breast cancer with metastisis. I put her in touch with Jon Sandifer at the Community Health Foundation in London and very much hope she will be helped in the way I have been.

In London, one of our friends lent us a flat which was a great help and avoided overcrowding the houses of Marian's brothers', especially as Gigi was with us, too. I saw my surgeon, John Cochrane, who was very impressed with my progress and with a normal full blood examination.

On our way back to Italy in April 1988, we stopped at Frankfurt to meet with Michio Kushi. He had been lecturing in a large building called "Pueblo," a well patronized health and social club with various health promoting activities, including squash courts. Michio examined me carefully and announced that in three months I would be well. He again urged us to write this book, promised to write a foreword and gave us the names of publishers in the United States who might publish it. He said I had no need of any further formal meetings, but should continue with the diet and way of life. This I have done with some minor modifications. During the summer of 1988, I began a course of Alexander postural rehabilitation. Some of our macrobiotic friends and counselors have commented on my posture and Ferro Ledvinka recommended the Alexander technique. We discovered that Fran Robinson, an enthusiastic and excellent Alexander teacher from London, (now living in Pontedera,) saw students in Florence twice a week. I managed with some difficulty, to get accepted as Ms. Robinson has more demands for tuition than she can satisfy. I had already known about the Alexander technique for many years and had sent patients in London to Dr. Wilfred Barlow, a well-known Alexander teacher who took over the leadership when the founder died. This brief account is based on information from Wilfred Barlow, Fran Robinson and an article by the Nobel prize winner, Nikolass Tinbergen, professor of animal behavior in the University of Oxford.

Frederick Matthias Alexander was born in Tasmania in 1869 and died in London in 1955. As a young actor he suddenly lost his voice. After orthodox medical treatment had failed to cure him, he became convinced that his problems were due to his posture and the misuse of his muscles. Without any scientific training or previous experience, he cured himself. He observed that the majority of people stand, sit and move in an inefficient manner. And so, as Tinbergen says, he became a kind of missionary and set out to teach, first actors, and then a variety of people, how to regain the proper use of their muscles.

The technique is based on exceptionally sophisticated observation and touch. It involves careful assessment and then gentle manipulation of the whole muscular system, according to the needs of each pupil. The number of lessons needed varies, but Fran recommends at least twenty-two lessons a week for five weeks and then one lesson a week for nine or ten weeks. Fran says that in my case it may take longer as I don't relax enough between lessons. Alexander teachers and successful pupils are convinced that many forms of under-performance and even physical and mental disorders can be helped, often to a surprising extent, by teaching the body to use its muscles efficiently. Since I am determined not only to defeat my cancer but also to become as fit as possible for my age, I decided to find out if the Alexander technique could help me. I'm now convinced that it played an important part in my rehabilitation.

Marian: Peter Hand, a sculptor, gives Hugh wood sculpture lessons in his house at Pontedera. After the first few sessions, Hugh was producing beautiful little bowls, and more recently, he produced a small statue. We are very pleased with these results, and intend to continue with our visits to Pontedera. While Hugh works with Peter, I walk and shop at one of the better health stores in Tuscany.

Hugh: According to Michio Kushi, I am now well, since it is many more than three months since I saw him. My fitness and sense of well-being support this, but I would feel happier if I had some objective evidence acceptable to my orthodox medical training that my cancer is disappearing or is at least inactive. Hilary Totah introduced me to macrobiotics at a key moment after my operation; some of my macrobiotic friends say it was no lucky chance but was determined by my karma. Marian tells me that the law of karma is described by Theosophists as the law of retribution or the law of cause and effect. As I understand it, when any action is performed a pre-ordained sequence of events is bound to occur, depending on the nature and strength of the action. However, Theosophists stress that this is not the same as fatalism and the loss of free will. We cannot escape our ruling destiny, but have the choice of two paths leading in that direction — we are free to choose the path leading to misery and despair, or that of salvation. I chose the latter!

The diet and way of life seem to suit me, and Marian's enthusiasm, the approval of my family and friends and the open-mindedness of my doctors have all helped. I cannot prove scientifically that the diet and the macrobiotic way of life have helped my body to reject the cancer, but no one can prove that they have not. I know, too, that a number of people have been praying for me, including members of my own family and the Australian Sisters of the Carmelite Order in Tavernelle, a neighboring commune in Chianti. I deeply appreciate the clean air and pure water, the warm sun, the peace and quiet of the Chianti countryside. In Chapter 2, I look at some of the possible factors involved in my recovery in more detail. John Cochrane, my surgeon, who brought his delightful family to see us two years ago, says that he doesn't know whether my recovery is due to macrobiotics or the will to live. I think it is due to both.

Marian: My hope and happiness increased rapidly as I watched Hugh's health improve. How important it is to have hope! I was reminded of Geoffrey De Purucker's book, *Wind of the Spirit*. I quote the following:

"As long as man has hope he does not despair. Weak or strong, it matters not; if he has hope, something to look forward to, if his inner spirit, the spiritual being within him, teaches him something of hope, he not only will never despair, but he will become a builder, a constructor, a worker with the universe, because he will move forwards, and this is altruism."

We are fortunate to have a macrobiotic East/West Center with its own food shop in Florence, plus another couple of good shops, and markets selling macrobiotic and vegetarian foods and supplies. I know there are others in many regions of Italy. Even our little town of Greve has a number of macrobiotic foods, much to our delight.

In Great Britain there is a lot of interest in whole foods and vegetarian and vegan diets. Macrobiotics is still not so well known as some of those who have heard of it think it is only a Japanese diet because of the use of several Japanese dried foods such as shiitake mushrooms, seaweed, and bancha or kukicha tea. Staying in Camden, North London, we had no difficulty in obtaining macrobiotic produce at Clearspring Natural Grocer, in Old Street. We also found a wide range of whole foods at the Bumblebee shops in Brecknock Road. It was good to see a number of supermarkets selling some of these foods, as well as many health stores in London and most towns in Britain. There are also a number of guests-houses prepared to cook the macrobiotic way and we found a useful guide at Genesis Books, *The Vegetarian Travel Guide 1991*.

Someone new to macrobiotics needs plenty of time to examine all the products carefully and read the small print. It takes longer to prepare the food thoughtfully and attractively, and cooking lessons are highly desirable if the food is to be prepared, cooked, served and eaten properly. The standard macrobiotic diet is for those of us who are fit. People with illnesses need to see a macrobiotic counselor who will recommend the appropriate adjustments for their condition. Hugh and I followed a carefully planned diet during the first two years after his diagnosis and received regular support from macrobiotic counselors.

Eating out was a problem at first, which we partly overcame by taking our own cooked food with us. Later, we would bring our whole rice or spaghetti to a restaurant and ask that it be cooked with their own vegetables and fish when available. Most of our friends are prepared to cook for us once they understand the basic diet, and many even enjoy the food. Now we are less fussy about our eating but still eat mainly at the macrobiotic restaurant when we are in Florence.

In April 1989, I was invited to tell my story at the Church in the Market Place at Isolotto near Florence. On a Sunday morning, I spoke to thirty or forty people under the sheds of the market, and answered questions afterwards. The Church resulted from a decision by two left-wing worker priests to continue their mission after a dispute with their bishop led to their removal from the parish church. For many years it has met every Sunday, winter and summer, in the open air. As far as I am concerned, it inspires its followers with a message far broader and more liberal than that of the official church. I was privileged to be allowed to take part and I felt very much at home there.

In the autumn of 1989, I gave a seminar at one of the Friday night dinner lectures sponsored by the Community Health Foundation in London. It was entitled "The Older and the Bolder." This went well, and we subsequently ran a workshop with the same title with Jon Sandifer in December, 1990, which was reasonably well attended.

When Michio Kushi was lecturing in Europe in 1989, he asked me to tell my story to some of the large audiences he attracted in Britain and Italy. Then he invited both of us to take part in the International Macrobiotic Summer Conference in August, 1990, at Amherst, near Boston, USA.

We duly set off by plane to Boston where we were met at the airport and driven by car to Amherst. The conference was held on the campus of the University during the summer vacation. We slept in a student's dormitory in a room with two bunks. We had our meals in the refectory, prepared by a team of experienced macrobiotic cooks with Wendy Rubin as head chef, assisted by several volunteers. The keynote lecture was given by John Robbins, author of the best seller *Diet for a New America*. This was an excellent start to the conference and I discuss it in more detail in Chapter 4.

There were several interesting seminars and lectures, and it was sometimes difficult to choose between them. We ourselves gave four seminars during the five days of the conference, telling our story and taking part in round table discussions. For the first time, Marian spoke in public. Her contributions to my story were much appreciated; there was even talk of having a session for wives, husbands and close friends of patients at future conferences.

We met many interesting people including Elaine Nussbaum whose own story is very moving, (Elaine Nussbaum, *Recovery*), and Dr. Sherry Rogers, one of the pioneers of environmental medicine and a confirmed macrobiotic, (Sherry Rogers, *Tired or Toxic*) who very kindly gave me a signed copy of her book.

It was a great pleasure to meet Michio and Aveline Kushi again, this time no longer as a client. They invited us to a very pleasant luncheon party to raise funds for the new Kushi Institute in Becket, now under construction. We also met William Dufty, author of the famous book on sugar, translated in several languages, (William Dufty, *Sugar Blues*) and Shizuko Yamamoto, who later gave me a most exciting shiatsu, in which she used not only her hands but also her bare feet! We met Shizuko again in New York, at the Macrobiotic Center which she founded. Here we gave a seminar at a dinner meeting which went very well.

At the beginning of November 1990, we flew to Berlin to attend the European Macrobiotic Congress. This was an unforgettable occasion for a number of reasons. It was held in the film studios of UFA, where some of the famous German films of the thirties were made. It is now a kind of commune where a number of people, mostly young, live and work to promote peace and ecological issues. Our excellent macrobiotic food was brought from the macrobiotic restaurant and served by volunteers. It was very moving to be in Berlin only a year or so after the wall was demolished, and a group from our congress held a session of prayer and mediation for peace where several people trying to cross the wall had been shot. Here they also planted an oak tree in remembrance.

The congress was fascinating. Many of the participants were actively engaged in some form of macrobiotic activity. The majority came from Europe, including Eastern Europe. We divided into committees to discuss various political, nutritional, and ecological issues. I joined the political group and was elected chairman. We chose to look at the congress itself and redefined its objectives and made some organizational proposals which were accepted by the congress. I describe the objectives in detail in Chapter 5. I was delighted to find many people had been thinking along similar lines to ourselves on the future of macrobiotics.

The story continues. We continue to follow the macrobiotic diet and way of life, though Marian still worries about what I consider to be minor deviations from the diet. For me, Michio's instructions and the various cookbooks provide a general guide and not a religious dogma to be followed grimly and precisely. I am convinced that fresh organically grown vegetables, free from pesticides and artificial fertilizers, are highly desirable. When our own supplies are not sufficient, Marian has managed to find sources for these in and around Florence, though they are more expensive than the commercially treated produce. Despite our frequent travels for lecturing, conferences, and family festivities, we hope to grow more of our own food in the future.

Our lives continue peacefully and happily — friends and family visit us, and we visit them. We still work part-time on our research project on old people, for which we seek additional funding. I am on the editorial board of our regional journal "Salute e Territorio" (Health and the Community), and also of our health district news sheet. We have worked on this book — still with a love/hate relationship with our word-processor, and plan another one on old people when this one is finished. We still swim two or three times a week, and also attend a local fitness class for the elderly.

In January, almost exactly four years after my original diagnosis of cancer of the pancreas, I saw my hospital specialists, Eric Beck and John Cochrane. I have just had a letter from them saying how good it was to see me "looking so well and full of vigor. A full blood count confirmed that all is well, and the serum and red cell folate levels are super-normal, doubtless, as Dr. Beck says "reflecting the macrobiotic diet."

Chapter 2
Recovery

Cancer of the pancreas is usually a rapid killer. It is an insidious tumor that frequently causes no pain or other symptoms in the early stages. Hence it is usually diagnosed late, and few people can expect to survive much more than six months after diagnosis. Even fewer survive one year and very few survive two years. It is now over five years since my diagnosis and I feel very fit, work hard, swim and attend keep-fit classes. I have more energy than I have had for years. The term "spontaneous regression" is used by doctors when a tumor appears to regress and they don't know why. Spontaneous regression is extremely rare in pancreatic cancer.

Some of the Medical Aspects of the Diet

I have followed the macrobiotic diet and way of life recommended by Michio Kushi reasonably faithfully — strictly in the first year, and with a few relaxations thereafter. Some, but not all, of these relaxations, were with Michio's permission. However, if I have any minor digestive upsets I treat them as a warning and return to a stricter observation of the diet to correct them. Michio's book *The Cancer Prevention Diet* deals more fully with the standard macrobiotic diet, which can be modified by an experienced counselor to suit a person's particular needs. Apart from a few details, the macrobiotic diet closely follows modern progressive, dietetic advice. Your own family doctor or your cancer surgeon will not necessarily be familiar with macrobiotics or even with orthodox modern dietetics. John Robbins says in his book, *Diet for a New America*, that in 1981 only 30 of the 125 medical schools in the United States had a single required course in nutrition, and that a recent Senate investigation revealed that the average doctor in the States received less than three hours training in nutrition during four years of medical school. This situation is very similar in the medical schools in Europe. We heard John lecture at the macrobiotic Summer Conference at Amherst, Massachusetts, in August 1990, and I have drawn heavily on his excellent and well documented book.

The situation is little better in the medical schools of Italy and Britain, the two countries I know best. All of us, including doctors, are exposed to the same propaganda extolling the virtues of meat and dairy products.

The Milk Marketing Board in Britain makes a special attempt to convince doctors. Some fifteen years ago, as an editor of a medical journal, I was offered a free holiday (which I refused) at one of their health establishments. The Meat Marketing Board in the States buys full page color advertisements in *J.A.M.A. (The Journal of the American Medical Association)* which is widely read by doctors.

It is incredible that it has taken us so long to realize the implications of information readily available in professional journals several years ago. In World War I the allied blockade of Denmark cut off all imports, and the government diverted all available grain to people instead of cattle. During the period of severest rationing, October 1917 to October 1918, the overall mortality rate was the lowest ever recorded. (1) During the German occupation of Norway in World War II meat was almost unobtainable. Once again the death rate from circulatory disease dropped dramatically. After the war, when Norwegians returned to their normal meat diet, the death rate rose accordingly. (2) Studies of populations living mainly on a vegetarian diet in Equador, the USSR and North Pakistan have revealed that they live longer and remain active in their eighties and nineties. Yet the popular image of long-haired, sandalled, vegetarian weaklings dies hard. John Robbins lists over twenty world-class athletes who were vegetarians. Yet our neighbors in Chianti still firmly believe that their menfolk need meat protein and animal fats to do a day's work on the land. This belief has no scientific basis, and I have seen no studies in the medical journals to support it.

In medical school, I was taught that animal proteins were first-class, and vegetable proteins were second-class and, therefore, inferior. This distinction, apparently based on experiments with rats, now appears to have been abandoned. Leading nutritionists state today that it is almost impossible to design a diet which provides adequate calories but which is deficient in protein. (John Robbins, *Diet for a New America*) It seems impossible to claim that one source of protein is superior to another, or that vegetarians have difficulty in obtaining protein. Obviously in the third world and among the very poor in our own societies, people are simply not getting enough food, therefore, not enough protein.

Some people are concerned about a lack of calcium in the macrobiotic diet. We were taught that cow's milk is an essential source of calcium, which prevents osteoporosis, particularly in older women. In fact, the main cause of osteoporosis has been found to be excessive protein! (3)

John Robbins quotes four other studies which show that even with high calcium intake, increased protein intake results in osteoporosis. High protein diets in general, and meat based diets in particular, lead to decrease in bone density and osteoporosis. (4)

There is also evidence that excess protein can lead to certain cancers According to Professor Campbell of Cornell University: "There is a strong correlation between dietary protein intake and cancer of the breast, prostate, pancreas and colon." (5)

Michio Kushi believes my pancreatic cancer was caused by eating too many eggs and too much chicken.

Nutrition, like immunology, genetics and molecular biology, is a relatively new, scientific discipline. As we have already said, it is comparatively neglected in most medical schools and few doctors are equipped to deal with it in practice. However, it is generally known that good wholesome food can support the immune system. It is perhaps less well known that heavily processed food contaminated with pesticides, high in animal protein and fat, cholesterol and refined sugars, can depress it. In recent years a number of books and articles in scientific journals have described the relationship between diet and immunity, but we are only at the beginning, and far more research is needed.

In the sixties we became conscious of the link between animal fats and heart disease. Saturated fat and cholesterol raise the blood cholesterol, favoring the formation of artherosclerosis, leading to a narrowing and blocking of arteries. When this occurs in the heart, the result is "coronary thrombosis," popularly known as "a heart attack." In the brain this gives rise to strokes. Heart attacks, stroke and cancer are the principle causes of death in the industrially developed countries. (Walford, R., *Maximum Life Span*). From 1963 to 1965, the International Atherosclerosis Project examined the arteries of over 20,000 autopsied bodies throughout the world. The results clearly showed a correlation between diets high in saturated fat and cholesterol and atherosclerosis, heart attacks and strokes. (Hausman, P., *Jack Sprat's Legacy — the Science and Politics of Fat and Cholesterol*). This and other studies caused consternation in the ranks of meat and dairy producers, who hastened to point out that coconuts, palm kernels and chocolate also contain cholesterol. This drew attention to the fact that these are the only plant foods significantly high in cholesterol.

During the past twenty years, a number of studies have demonstrated that atherosclerosis results from a dietary intake of saturated fat and cholesterol. The dairy, meat and poultry industries in industrialized countries have vigorously contested these findings, and financed several studies attempting to disprove it, but were not successful. They demonstrated that carnivorous animals do not get atherosclerosis however much meat they eat, but failed to show that human beings are among them. Of all the factors known to be involved in heart disease — obesity, lack of exercise, refined sugar, coffee, smoking, raised blood pressure, lack of dietary fiber — saturated fat and cholesterol are by far the most important.

Although the main outlines are clear, research continues in this area, and there are conflicting opinions on the details of the processes involved. I am certainly not equipped to deal with the technicalities in this field and anyone especially interested in this important subject should consult one of the recent books published. For our immediate purpose, it is enough to know that there are basically two kinds of dietary fat: saturated and unsaturated. Most of the fat in red meat, lard, butter, cow's milk, hard cheeses and poultry is saturated. These are invariably accompanied by cholesterol. On the other hand, the fats in grains, vegetables and fruit are unsaturated and easier to assimilate, with the exception of palm and coconut oil. Polyunsaturated fat is the least dense form of unsaturated fat and hence the easiest to assimilate. A molecule is said to be "saturated" when all its available carbon bonds are occupied by hydrogen atoms; unsaturated fats have more carbon bonds left free. (Kushi, Michio and Cottrell Martha, in *AIDS, Macrobiotics and Natural Immunity*).

Macrobiotic counselors recommend that almost all vegetables and fruits be lightly cooked. Ideally, they should be home grown or obtained from a reliable organic grower. All locally grown fruit and vegetables are acceptable with the exception of the nightshade or solanaceous family which includes potatoes, tomatoes, peppers, aubergine, and courgettes — introduced to Europe comparatively recently. All tropical plants, fruits, palm and coconut oils are also excluded. These are all regarded as extremely yin in the yin/yang classification, and are to be avoided.

John Robbins has carefully collected a mass of evidence to support his case, although his family is said to own the largest, multinational company manufacturing ice cream in the world! I have on selecting a small part of this evidence, attempted to show that the macrobiotic diet, though originally based on Oriental traditional medicine, is entirely consistent with these relatively recent discoveries in the field of nutrition. It can no longer be dismissed as quaint Eastern folklore without relevance for us today.

The Biology of Hope

While I am convinced that the macrobiotic diet has played an important role in my case, I believe that many other factors have also had a share in my recovery. These I have grouped under Norman Cousins' title, *The Biology of Hope*. (6)

For many years Norman Cousins was the editor of the Saturday Review. He describes in *Anatomy of an Illness* how he cured himself of a serious collagen illness, a disease of the connective tissue. In 1970 he resigned from his editorship and, although he had no medical qualification, was invited to join the faculty of the Department of Psychiatry and Biobehavioral Science at UCLA (the University of California, Los Angeles). Here he taught and assisted in research in the growing field of psychoneuroimmunology. (PNI). For some time a number of researchers outside mainstream immunology have been observing the influence of various psychological processes on immune responses. Gradually, psychologists, neurophysiologists and immunologists have begun to see the fundamental links between their various fields. Out of this realization the relatively new science of psychoneuroimmunology (PNI) has emerged.

At the Seventh International Congress of Immunology in Berlin, (August, 1989), there were over 160 papers dealing with interactions between the immune and the nervous systems. Psychoneuroimmunology "represents a much more differentiated, more finely tuned articulation of disease and healing processes, increasingly dissolving the three long-standing dualisms of mind and body, body and environment, individual and population. For the first time, medicine is equipped with a discourse capable of formulating very specific correlations between (i) the patient's bodily experienced meaning and (ii) conditions or states of the medical body, the body that figures in the research and clinical practices of medicine. (8)

We have long realized that anxiety, depression and stress can have a direct effect on our physiology. Hans Selye made a great contribution in this field. Many years ago I heard him lecture, in English, in his old university in Prague. Faced with a patient who has a terminal illness, at least in the terms of Western medicine, a doctor has a difficult choice. Should he tell the patient the truth as he sees it? Or should he compromise and leave him a modicum of hope? American doctors say that their lawyers advise them to "tell the truth, the whole truth and nothing but the truth," in order to protect themselves from possible lawsuits from patients' families. Yet in doing so they may be lowering their patient's resistance and making recovery less likely. No doctor can possibly give a precise estimate of survival time, and many of us have always tried to avoid anything in the nature of a death sentence, without departing too far from the facts as we see them.

My own doctors at the Whittington Hospital never said, in so many words, that my illness was terminal. Maybe they knew I would look up the prognosis in the medical literature and, anyway, I never asked. When I learned that I could expect to live two to six months from the date of diagnosis, this only confirmed what I already knew, so I was not particularly shocked. However, at this stage, it never occurred to me that I could do anything to extend my life, and I accepted the verdict of orthodox medicine without question.

When I first read that some people believed that macrobiotics could help the body to reject cancer, it was a revelation. I certainly wasn't intellectually convinced, but perhaps there was something I could do. Here was hope, however slim, and what did I have to lose? Looking back, the first result of our decision to try macrobiotics — a decision my family and friends fully supported — was the feeling that I had regained control of the situation. At this stage this could have been completely illusory. But I was doing something; whether it would lead to success or failure, I didn't know.

In my interview with Edward Esko, my first meeting with a macrobiotic counselor, I was conscious of something else.

Edward's complete certainty that I would recover came across to both Marian and myself and gave us real hope for the first time since my diagnosis. Hence, I believe that Edward began my recovery and I told him so when we met again at the 1990 Macrobiotic Summer Conference at Amherst.

I can't prove scientifically that the renewal of hope had a direct effect on my immune system. Although the science of psychoneuroimmunology is only in its infancy, it could provide some exciting scientific findings in the next few years. A number of studies carried out by the psychoneuroimmunology unit in the University of California have clearly demonstrated that positive emotions have a positive effect on the immune system. On the other hand, emotional distress results in negative immune functions. This latter finding was more evident in older people, in whom the relationship between psychological factors and immune function seems stronger than in younger people. However, the immune systems of older people in good health are as functional as, and in some ways superior to, those of healthy persons half their age. The immune systems of both old and young were comparably enhanced by vigorous physical exercise.

This work has confirmed by belief that hope, combined with a macrobiotic diet and life-style, played a vital role in my recovery. When I see patients who have been told that they have terminal cancer, I naturally tell them of this work and my own experience, but I am careful to remind them that we are all different. There is no guarantee that they will have the same results I did, but there is always hope!

Lifestyle

Macrobiotic counselors always stress that macrobiotics does not consist only of the diet. The English word *diet* derives from the medieval Latin "diaetare" which, according to the *Oxford English Dictionary*, means "to live according to a certain plan" and is not limited to food consumption. Since traditional Eastern medicine regards all illness as a lack of harmony between the individual and nature as a whole, it seeks to help the body restore that harmony. This should be easy for those of us living in a calm peaceful corner of the Chianti hills, surrounded by woods and birds and wild animals provided the hunters leave us in peace. We have consciously tried to draw closer to the wildlife, have built artificial nests for the birds and bats and homes for the hedgehogs. We walk in the woods, though with all our other activities, not often enough.

I have exercised more regularly since my illness. I was never a keen swimmer, but now find great satisfaction in swimming. I miss it when we can't find time for it or when we are traveling. In the first year we tried to follow Michio's injunction to reduce traveling to a minimum, but I pointed out that a major part of our traveling at that time consisted in trying to meet with him a various parts of Europe for consultations!

Macrobiotic counselors strongly recommend the use of natural fabrics. Clothing made from artificial fiber is believed to reduce the flow of energy between the skin and the natural environment, while natural fiber allow the energy to flow freely (cotton or linen should be worn next to the skin.) We try to follow this advice as far as possible. We also try to avoid chemically produced cosmetics, soaps and shampoos. Natural vegetable products are now widely available.

Since my illness I have drawn closer to family and friends. This is not necessarily the result of macrobiotics, but its general philosophy has helped. My relationship with Marian has deepened and strengthened, and she has willingly and cheerfully taken part in every aspect of our new life, including valiantly attempting to master the mysteries of our new word processor and all the trials and tribulations of producing a book. Without her love and active support, it would have all been much more difficult.

1. Hindehede, Mikkel. *The Effect of Food Restrictions during War of Mortality in Copenhagen.*

2. Strom A. And Jensen R.A. *Mortality From Circulatory Disease in Norway.*

3. John N. et al.,*Effect of Level of Protein Intake on Urinary and Fecal Calcium Retention.*

4. Altschuler, S. *Dietary Protein and Calcium Loss: a Review.*

5. Lang, S. *Diet and Disease.*

6 Cousins, Norman. *Head First — The Biology of Hope.*

7. Booth, Roger. *Psychoneuroimmunology.*

8. Leven, D.M. And Solomon, G.F. Esalen Institute. (non-dated paper)

9. Cousins, Norman. Ibid

Chapter 3
A General Look at Macrobiotics

Since I believe that macrobiotics and the macrobiotic way of life has played an important role in my recovery from pancreatic cancer, it seems reasonable to find out how this has come about. Modern macrobiotics is based on traditional Oriental medicine and Ted Kaptchuk's book is invaluable as an introduction to Eastern traditional medicine as a whole. (1)

Apart from the bare essentials of elementary acupuncture technique, the theoretical depth and clinical potential of a complex medical system are almost completely unknown to doctors in the West. For the most part, traditional Eastern medicine is seen as a quaint survivor of folklore and magic. Modern Western scientific medicine is seen as providing the only source of truth in the field of health. A growing number of people in the West question this view, partly because Western medicine, despite its very real achievements, has failed to prevent or cure the chronic degenerative conditions which cause most deaths and disability in our societies. A minority has turned to the East, seeing Eastern philosophy and medicine as more mysterious, more spiritual, more holistic and therefore more "true" than Western medicine. This mistaken approach tends to turn a rational discipline — albeit based on premises vastly different from our own into a religious faith. Dr. Kaptchuk sees Chinese medicine as "a coherent and independent system of thought and practice that has been developed over two millennia. It is, however, based on the philosophy, theory and practice of civilizations completely different from our own. The main difference in perception and labelling between traditional Chinese medicine and Western biomedicine is the understanding of the relation/identity of psyche and soma." (2)

I have been actively looking for information about lifestyle and cancer since my own diagnosis five years ago. I now realize that many alternative approaches to cancer had appeared before this, as well as a considerable amount of research into the effect of the mind on physiological processes. But little of this has been known to the general public or to doctors, who, if they knew about it at all, regarded it as unproven folk-lore, and of little interest.

In February 1990, an international conference was organized in London by the *British Journal of Hospital Medicine,* generally regarded as a conservative journal, on the subject of "Cancer and the Mind." Cancer specialists, psychiatrists, psychologists, immunologists, sociologists, complementary practitioners and patients — in all over 500 doctors and nurses — attended. This shows the enormous interest of the orthodox medical profession in this subject and makes the need for extending the dialogue between complementary medicine and orthodox Western medicine increasingly necessary. Not all the speakers agreed with one another, but a majority seemed to accept that behavior and attitude could affect the onset or progress of cancer. Diet was not discussed at the conference but several speakers made observations highly relevant to our work in macrobiotics.

A cancer patient, Dr. Dennison, quoted Carl Roger's definition of a good therapist. He defines three essential qualities of a person centered approach: 'genuineness'; (no professional front or personal facade), 'acceptance,' (unconditional positive regard towards the patient) and 'empathetic understanding.' He says, "This kind of sensitive, active listening is extremely rare in our lives. We think we listen, but very rarely do we listen with real understanding and true empathy. Yet listening of this very special kind is one of the most potent forces for change that I know."

Many doctors would find this kind of listening extremely difficult, and perhaps our failure to listen to our patients is causing many people to turn to complementary medicine. Macrobiotic counselors find it easier intuitively to listen in this way.

Patrick Peitroni, the founder of the Holistic Medical Society in Britain, made an interesting point on the shift from what he called 'masculine' interventions — chemotherapy, radiotherapy and surgery — to the 'feminine' therapies — listening, caring, holding, touching, massaging and imagery. This strengthened my belief that more women should become macrobiotic counselors, and not see their only place as the kitchen. Dr. Pietroni further suggested that all of us working in this area should ask ourselves three questions:

1. Do our interventions affect the life of cancer patients?
2. Do these interventions affect their long-term survival?
3. Does the long-term practice of these techniques prevent the occurrence of cancer?

In macrobiotics fully accurate answers to these questions are not yet available. Clearly there are far more factors involved than in most medical, clinical, trials and research is far more complicated. Nevertheless, we have to go on trying to answer these questions. Until we do my medical colleagues will not take us seriously.

Several speakers believed that some form of group psychotherapy can facilitate and reinforce the development of a fighting spirit and defeat the feeling of helplessness experienced by cancer patients. I know some macrobiotic counselors are interested in humanistic psychotherapy and are already using some of the techniques involved. It would be interesting to offer cancer patients the opportunity to participate in a support group, in addition to giving them diet and lifestyle suggestions. This would probably only be possible in a center with many cancer patients, and might require the help of a psychologist trained in group therapy. If behavior therapy can change people's attitudes and lifestyles, such groups could also have a preventive role.

Dr. Moorey, a lecturer in psychological medicine at the Royal Marsden Hospital, quoted Albert Schweitzer as saying that the greatest discovery of any generation is that human beings can change their lives by altering their attitudes of mind. The medicine I was taught in a London medical school fifty years ago was concerned mainly with defining disease categories, disclosing their pathology, and determining a precise cause and cure for a specific disease. The mind was barely mentioned. I created a sensation by asking to learn about psychiatry, which proved to be quite impossible in the London Hospital Medical College in those days. Our teaching was firmly based on the Newtonian, Cartesian mechanistic approach. Eastern medicine is concerned with the physiology and psychology of each individual patient. All available information from a person's history and a detailed examination is used to reveal what is called a "pattern of disharmony." This approach is essentially holistic, no single finding can be interpreted without relating it to the whole. It is based on the traditional concept of yin and yang.

Yin and yang are neither physical forces nor material entities. They are simply convenient labels to explain the continuous movement of constant change, in Marxist terminology, the interpenetration of opposites, and the relationship of all things to one another and the whole. (3)

Yin is the name given to energy or movement that is expanding. Yang is the name given to energy or movement that is contracting. Yin is associated with cold, rest, passivity, darkness, plants, female. Yang is associated with heat, stimulation, activity, light and animals. All things have a yin aspect and a yang aspect, including illnesses.

Ki, the life force, flows through the meridians and forms the basis of all acupuncture and shiatsu treatment. As far as I know, it has not yet been possible to detect or measure Ki or define the meridians scientifically, though the anesthetic and analgesic actions of acupuncture have been demonstrated. Research workers in Rumania, Britain and the United States, however, claim to have demonstrated the presence of "...magnetic fields which can act therapeutically by facilitating the communication between aberrant cells and adjacent normal cells, which can therefore bring about a return to normality." (4)

Macrobiotics has adopted the philosophy and general approach of traditional Eastern medicine, but not all of its applications in practice. Ron Kotzsch, in his excellent book, describes in some detail how macrobiotics has evolved over the years. Any reader who wants more information on the history of macrobiotics and, in particular, the fascinating — and sometimes surprising — lives of the founding fathers, should read Ron Kotzsch's book. (5)

The general Japanese diet in the mid-19th century appears to have closely resembled a macrobiotic diet. Cattle were bred for work, not for meat, and dairy products were unkown. When, in 1859, the American ambassador asked for a cow to provide milk for his tea, the Japanese diplomats were incredulous. Despite this, the Japanese rapidly adopted Western ways. In 1871, the first German physicians arrived to teach and to practice Western medicine and surgery. By 1883 traditional medicine was banned, and only Western medicine permitted.

Although George Ohsawa is generally regarded as the founder of macrobiotics, Kotzsch has chosen Ekken Kaibara (1630-1716) as its earliest forerunner. Kaibara traveled widely and wrote books on botany, geography, herbal remedies and morals. At the age of eighty-three he wrote a book which was translated into English with the title *Japanese Secrets of Good Health*. In Chapter One, he says "...it is only natural that one who has learned health preservation and who applies it, will become strong in body, will shirk off all diseases, will live to the age Providence meant him to live to, and enjoy it too..." Sickness, like health, is something that mankind creates. Quoting the Tao Te Ching, Kaibara notes that "One's life is in one's own hands." Perhaps the only part of his advice unacceptable to use today lies in his strict rules for sexual intercourse. Kotzsch notes humorously, "If all the restrictions are observed one may indulge only on cloudless, overcast evenings during the new moon in a thatched cave opening to the northwest." As far as I know, this recommendation is not followed by any of our macrobiotic friends today.

If we accept Kaibara as the grandfather of macrobiotics, it seems reasonable to call Doctor Sagen Ishizuka the founder of the modern discipline. Born in 1860, in a period of rapid expansion and modernization, he felt that much of great value in traditional medicine was being lost. He set out to revive it and present it in a modern scientific form. It was on this foundation that Ohsawa and others built.

Ishizuka studied both Oriental and Western medicine and qualified as a doctor. At the age of twenty-eight he became a physician in the Japanese army. He developed a chronic renal condition which Western medicine failed to cure. He began to experiment with his diet and abandoned meat and dairy products and ate mainly brown rice, and recovered. At one time he lived for a month on only sweet potatoes. He also embarked on anthropological and chemical studies and read the Western scientific journals. He published his magnum opus *A Chemical Nutritional Theory of Long Life* in 1897, at the age of thirty seven. He cites countless experiments of his own and others to support his theories, determined to provide a "respectable" scientific explanation for them. In the following year he produced for the general public, a practical handbook on diet which wen through twenty three editions. His fame grew in leaps and bounds and he had to limit the number of patients he saw to 100 a day! Letters addressed to "Dr. Miso Soup, Tokyo" reached him. In 1908, a group of his supporter formed the "Food Cure Society," in effect the first macrobiotic organization.

Several years after the founding of this society, a young student, Yukikazu Sakurazawa, came across a book by Ishizuka. The young man was later known in the West as George Ohsawa. He was born in Kyoto in 1893. From about 1923 until his death in 1966, the history of macrobiotics is virtually the story of Ohsawa's life and works. Both his mother and brother died from pulmonary tuberculosis and he himself contracted the disease. Given little hope by Western medicine he followed Ishizuka's teaching and recovered. Until the age of thirty he was a successful businessman and travelled widely in the West. In 1923 the Tokyo fire and earthquake destroyed the headquarters of his firm and he lost his job. He turned to the Shoku-Yo movement, where he seems to have rapidly become a leading figure. He took over publications and wrote and spoke widely, drawing chiefly from Ishizuka.

Although Ohsawa never realized his dream of a worldwide macrobiotic revolution, he inspired many young men and women by his lectures and seminars. Aveline Kushi still speaks of him with affection and admiration and is planning a celebration in 1993 to mark the centenary of his birth. Some of his students, including Michio and Aveline Kushi, and Herman and Cornelia Aihara, went on to carry the torch of the revival of traditional medicine in the United States and later throughout the world.

Michio came to the United States in 1949 at the age of twenty three, intending to study international law and world peace. Tomoko Yokoyama, later to be known as Aveline Kushi, was studying with George Ohsawa in Japan at the time, and she first became aware of Michio Kushi due to the interesting letters the young man was sending to her teacher. She was so impressed with these letters that she decided to join Michio in the United States, and she made the journey in 1951. Shortly after, Herman and Cornelia Aihara also arrived in the United States.

In the mid-sixties, the Kushis moved to Boston, which became the main focus of macrobiotics on the East coast, while the Aiharas developed increasing activity in the West. The story of their struggles is told vividly by Aveline Kushi in her autobiography, *Aveline: The Life and Dream of the Woman Behind Macrobiotics Today.* (6) Michio developed his own approach and steadily liberalized Ohsawa's dietary recommendations. He wrote, lectured, and taught continuously, and gradually trained and inspired a whole number of men and women, many of whom have made their own contributions and developed centers in Europe and in other parts of the United States. Aveline, as well as being involved in the organization, became a leading exponent of macrobiotic cooking and has written several excellent books on the subject. She told us once in one of her cooking classes, that the last thing she intended to do when she was young was to spend her life in the kitchen! Marian and I were entertained in the Kushi house in Brookline, Massachusetts, during our recent visit to the United States. The Kushi Institute has now moved from Boston to Becket, Massachusetts.

Now, some thirty years after Ohsawa first presented macrobiotics in his lectures in New York, considerable progress has been made. There are two major educational centers (Vega and the Kushi Institute), which some 300 students attend every year. The worldwide macrobiotic directory of 1984 listed some 175 "macrobiotic centers, friends and businesses" in Canada and the United States, 150 certified teachers and counselors, and three macrobiotic journals. The annual summer conference in New England attracts about 600 people.

In Europe the small beginnings, stimulated by Ohsawa, virtually came to a standstill after his death. In 1972, Bill Tara, who had been managing the macrobiotic natural food company, Erewhon, in Boston settled in London and started activity from his home. In 1974, he and Peter Bradford set up Sunwheel Foods. By 1976, they had sufficient support to found the Community Health Foundation in a large five-story Victorian school in Old Street, where it is today. In 1981, Bill Tara returned to the United States to direct the Kushi Institute and Denny Waxman came to London for two years to organize the Community Health Foundation. Since then it has been run first by Jon Sandifer and now by Simon Brown, who have both developed the activities of the Center with considerable success.

The only other center we know personally is in Florence, in Via Serragli. The East West Center was set up by Ferro Ledvinka in 1983 in a 16th century building previously used as a student commune. The Center organizes lectures and courses and provides macrobiotic counseling and shiatsu. The macrobiotic restaurant, Santommasio, is in Via Romana. There are other centers in Turin, Genoa, Milan, Pesaro and smaller groups in several other cities in Italy.

With the emerging of new macrobiotic centers in Russia and Eastern Europe and the opening of the new home for the Kushi

Institute in Becket, a new era seems to be opening for macrobiotics.

1. Kaptchuk, T. *The Web That Has No Weaver.*

2. Ots, Thomas. *The Angry Liver, The Anxious Heart and the Melancholy Spleen.*

3. Levins, R. and Lewontin, R. *The Dialectical Biologist.*

4. Oldfield and Coghill:. *The Dark Side of the Brain.*

5. Kotzch, R. *Macrobiotics — Yesterday and Today.*

6. Kushi, Aveline and Alex Jack. *Aveline: The Life and Dream of the Woman Behind Macrobiotics Today.*

Chapter 4
Macrobiotics and a Wider View

"One should not walk through the world wearing blinders."
— Albert Einstein

Macrobiotics is at a crossroads today. What does it mean to its followers? For some of us it has provided a lifeline when orthodox medicine offered no hope, and no effective system of prevention. For others it is a retreat from modern Western civilization, a protest against the worst excesses of consumerism, against the destruction of the environment for financial gain, against violence and war. For still others it is the "journey to the East" which the "flower people" followed in the sixties. They happily embrace traditional Japanese philosophy, perhaps the Buddhist religion, Japanese customs and even dress. But others, less concerned with the East, appear to be simply seeking a life as close to nature as possible, growing their own food organically, making their own soy derivatives, baking their own bread, and perhaps making their own clothes. Some reject Western science and medicine completely, and turn to magic and mysticism. They show little concern or responsibility for the wider society, and are engrossed only with their own salvation and that of their immediate companions. Others seem to be making macrobiotics a substitute for religion. We are in no position to sneer at such approaches. We share much of the desire to reject the consumeristic society and also seek to live as close to nature as we can. But surely this is not enough.

We all have a responsibility to work with others for peace and for a world free from exploitation. That Marian and I are not alone in this belief became clear at the last meeting of the European Macrobiotic Congress in Berlin in November, 1990, attended mainly by people active in some sphere of macrobiotics.

Perhaps those of us who have come to macrobiotics with an "incurable," life-threatening illness can be expected to have a different perspective. We are not necessarily travelers on the "journey to the East" or life in a rural community. We have not all rejected Western science and medicine though we may have many criticisms and reservations. We are profoundly grateful for the help we have received, but still ask: "Where is macrobiotics going?" In the foreseeable future only a minority of citizens in any Western country will seek to join "the journey to the East" or be attracted to rural communes. They will remain a relatively select in-group, for the most part, middle class. This is surely not what George Ohsawa dreamed of, and I am convinced that Michio Kushi has far wider plans for the new center at Becket. Macrobiotics faces a major challenge and a great opportunity. In reviving traditional medicine, George Ohsawa discovered lessons of supreme importance and relevance to Western society today. In no country is this yet realized and perhaps it's not always fully realized in macrobiotic circles.

It is important that we find new ways of continuing the dialogue between macrobiotics, traditional Eastern medicine and Western medicine. Inevitably Western doctors and their patients will ask, "Does it work?" and despite many anecdotal accounts of personal recovery, macrobiotics has yet to provide the evidence that could satisfy Western medical science. Kaptchuk suggests that perhaps some such evidence already exists. After the victory of the communists in China in 1949, the leadership decided to take a fresh look at traditional Chinese medicine. It appears that thousands of trials and experiments were carried out during the fifties.

In 1958, the Chinese communist party became convinced that traditional medicine worked in practice, and despite the Party's lack of success in the political and economic fields, it was not necessarily wrong in this. The government decided to give traditional and modern Western medicine equal rights, often in the same hospital. Patients were offered the choice of which system to consult. I do not know if this continues today. Perhaps with the enthusiasm for a consumer orientated market displayed by the present leadership, the pendulum will have swung back in favor of Western medicine. Yet the reports of these clinical studies should still exist, even if expressed in terms and methodology completely foreign to Western medicine, and could well be extremely informative.

"There is hardly a field in all of historical scholarship of which we know so little as the development of Chinese medical thought." (1)

This probably applies equally to Japanese traditional medicine, although a growing interest in acupuncture and shiatsu in the West has led to what seems too often to be a superficial study of Ki (or in the Chinese form Ch'i) and the meridians. Meridians are "energetic circuits" on which acupuncture, shiatsu and moxibustion are based. Moxibustion involves applying heat at the acupuncture points. The heat is produced by igniting mugwort (artemesia vulgaris) which can be purchased in already prepared sticks. Many unsuccessful attempts have been made in the West to detect some kind of anatomical structure involved, or define some measurable magnetic force. This is surely a potentially fruitful field for cooperative research into the vast literature on Eastern medicine, so far mostly in Chinese or Japanese. But traditional Eastern medicine has far more to offer than acupuncture and shiatsu, useful as these techniques are. Macrobiotics has inherited this approach and is applying it in day to day practice.

Much of this Eastern thinking is highly relevant to the problems facing health care today. In the macrobiotic view, life consists of two forces, yin and yang, dialectically opposed and in constant motion. Each individual is unique and cannot be seen as an entity separate from his total environment. Ill health is seen as an imbalance between the individual and nature. Western medicine, on the other hand, concentrates on the disease and tries to probe it at every level including cellular and molecular. This approach developed from the Newtonian-Cartesian science which saw the human body as an extremely complex machine, and is responsible for the very real technological advances in recent years. It, too, often fails to see the individual patient as a whole — as a unique organic being, in his social, emotional and physical setting. Marxists have frequently pointed this out, and it would be interesting to promote discussion between macrobiotics and biologists who have used the approach of dialectical materialism in their work. (2)

I am not competent to discuss the recent advances of research in physics and allied disciplines, and I have only the haziest notions of relativity and quantum mechanics. However, even a casual reading of some books and articles on popular science suggests that much of the medical science I was taught fifty years ago is probably incompatible with recent research, and that some of the concepts of Eastern medicine and macrobiotics begin to seem less improbable.

A profound crisis is developing in health care in Europe and North America. Medicine based on high-powered, sophisticated technology is producing steadily soaring costs, while at the same time, increasing numbers of people are becoming aware of the shortcomings of our health care systems and their conceptual framework. (3)

A new global view of society in which political, economic, social and environmental factors are intimately interwoven is developing rapidly. Western medical science, with its emphasis on high technology, with the exclusion of disease prevention and health promotion, risks being left behind.

Has macrobiotics a world view? In his lectures Michio Kushi implies that it has. But some of our friends in macrobiotics seem reluctant to admit it, and appear to see only dangers if macrobiotics enters the wider political arena. Yet many of our aims are already political — clean air, pure water, wholesome uncontaminated food, and environment free from violence, a world without war. These cannot be realized without political action. The new objectives of the International Macrobiotic Assembly accept this challenge and represent an important step forward for macrobiotics:

1. To provide a forum for discussion of macrobiotic ideas and practice.

2. To evolve projects at an international level relevant to macrobiotic activity.

3. To collaborate in joint projects with other organizations in social action in the field of health and ecology.

4. To provide networking and support for macrobiotic activists and organizations in each country.

5. To stimulate and support the growth of macrobiotic activities in countries and areas where they are not yet developed.

Today there is a growing consensus on what constitutes a healthy diet. Sir Richard Doll, former Regius Professor of medicine at Oxford, summed it up as long ago as 1982: "Whether the object is to avoid cancer, coronary heart disease, hypertension, diabetes, diverticular disease, duodenal ulcer or constipation, there is broad agreement among research workers that the type of diet that is least likely to cause disease is one that provides a high proportion of calories in whole grain cereals, vegetables and fruit; provides most of its animal protein in fish and poultry; limits the intake of fats, and, if oils are to be used, gives preference to liquid vegetable oils; includes very few dairy products, eggs, and little refined sugar." (4)

It is remarkable how close this is to a macrobiotic diet.

Four years later in 1984, the British Medical Association — not always in the vanguard of progress — said in a report by its Board of Science and Education:

"The Ministry of Agriculture, Fisheries and Food will wish to support the food industry... Present policies artificially raise consumption of either potentially harmful products, such as sugar, whole fat milk and butter, or less healthy products such a white bread." (5)

Some Kushi Institutes and macrobiotic centers are beginning to invite speakers from other organizations and disciplines. For example, John Robbins, author of the best selling *Diet for a New America*, gave the keynote lecture at the 1990 Macrobiotic Summer Conference at Amherst, Massachusetts, which aroused a great deal of interest and discussion among the participants. I hope this example will be followed in other places, and speakers will be invited from the many areas of common interest — ecology, pollution, traffic, pesticides, organic agriculture, food additives, bird and animal sanctuaries, health promotion and prevention of illness, and scientific research — particularly in psychoneurology and immunology.

Despite their immense power, the multinationals are extremely sensitive to public opinion and any adverse criticism which can directly affect sales. This needs to be carried out on a mass scale, and will demand cooperation with other like-minded organizations and individuals. Of course, this is "dabbling in politics," but we must never forget that any effective action is "political" whether we like it or not. Even passivity is political action, in support of the status quo.

Once we convince any government of the political necessity to do something about the issues regarding food, ecology, and pollution, mass pressure could bring about legislation which could greatly reduce, if not abolish, the worst of the abuses. Such changes will not come about spontaneously. The politicians have got to be told that these new policies are vote-winners. In the development of mass pressure we all have a part to play, and macrobiotics can have an important role. We cannot afford to stand aside.

We have met few women in a leading role in macrobiotics with the obvious exceptions of Aveline Kushi and Shizuko Yamamoto in New York. Yet macrobiotic counseling seems to be ideally suited to the special skills and gifts of women, whose activities should surely not be solely confined to the kitchen, however essential and exciting the art of macrobiotic cooking may be. As men took control of the medical establishment in the West, women were gradually excluded from their traditional roles in healing. Midwives were replaced by obstetricians, medical cookery and herbalism were absorbed in the academic fields of pharmacy, dietetics and botany — fields dominated mainly by men. Midwives who had been doctors and teachers of other women became assistants to obstetricians and only worked on their own with the very poor, who could not afford a doctor. Women became "ancillaries" — in ancient Greece the handmaidens to the Gods. As the male expert, legitimized by regulations and medical schools which excluded women, took over all organized health care, women lost control over their own health. As early as 1666, Margaret Cavendish wrote: "For though the Muses, Graces and Sciences are all of feminine gender, yet they were more esteemed in former ages than they are now; nay, could it be done handsomely, they would turn them all from Females into Males; so great is grown the self-conceit of the Masculine, and the disregard of the Female Sex." Let us determine that macrobiotics will restore women to a leading role in health care.

1. Porkert, M. *The Theoretical Foundations of Chinese Medicine.* (see Forward by Nathan Sivin.)

2. Levins, Richard and Lewontin, Richard. *The Dialectical Biologist.*

3. Dossey, L. *Space, Time and Medicine.*

4. Cannon, G. *The Politics of Food*

5. Cannon, G. Ibid.

Chapter 5
The Older the Bolder

Granny learned to dance at eighty-two
A really odd type thing to do,
And when she'd learned both tap and ballet,
She changed her name from Maud to Sally.

She said: "Till now I've done things right,
I've never stayed up all the night,
Or learned a great magician's trick,
Or eaten cake until I'm sick.

I was too busy, don't you see,
To ever really just be me."

— Nanette Newman, "My Granny"
Quoted by Bernice Martin

After I began to believe my cancer was in remission, I realized that I felt fitter and more energetic than I had for years. If this was the result of the macrobiotic diet and lifestyle, could it help others of my age who didn't have cancer? Further, without the threat of a death sentence, would any of my fellow senior citizens be prepared to change the habits of a lifetime?

Many years ago, I heard of a club started by the novelist C.R. Vevinson called "The Older the Bolder." I never knew any details, but I believe the club organized adventure holidays for older people, and the name stayed in my mind. Looking back over my patients, relatives and friends, I realized that old people fall roughly into two categories: those who see old age as a threat and those who see it as a challenge. Why is there such an enormous difference between different people of the same age? Why do some people lose their autonomy and independence and others not?

This is the area our research project seeks to explore. Shortly before my illness, our health district (which covers six provinces of the Chianti zone,) planned research into the relative risk of the factors involved in the loss of autosufficiency in old people in the area. In the first phase we intend to organize meetings of small groups of old people in two of our provinces, one truly rural and one closer to Florence and more urban.

Our project is based on a number of hypotheses; for example, that each individual is unique, that there are probably major differences between old people in different settings, and that old people themselves may provide information in small groups that has not emerged in the many traditional questionnaires which have been carried out in several places. We have been promised funding for our pilot survey by the EEC, and now seek further financing to complete the project.

In the past 200 years, the demographic profile of most countries, including Britain, has been completely transformed. (1)

Instead of populations consisting mainly of young adults and children, in Britain one-third of the population is now over the age of fifty and nearly a fifth over sixty. On the average, girls born in 1986 can expect to live to the age of seventy-eight, six years longer than their brothers. This change is mainly due to decreases in the birth rate and death rate. Both have many causes. Curative medicine may have played a part in prolonging life and vaccination has helped to reduce the incidence of the killer infections of childhood, but the death rate had begun to decline long before these became widely available, and appears to be due mainly to improved diet and living and working conditions. We can expect the death rate at all ages to decrease steadily in the last decade of the millennium. In 1981 only eleven in each 1000 of the population in Britain were age eighty-five or more, but by the year 2001 some seventeen in each 1000 will be eighty-five or older. Inevitably those over eighty-five are more likely to become dependent on care, but as Prof. Jeffreys points out "A technologically innovative and ingenious society such as ours ought to be able to sustain such a proportion of dependents even if they were all, as they clearly are not, in need of tending day in and day out." However, this won't happen automatically, and the community services for the elderly today are far from universally adequate, and vary greatly from place to place, and country to country.

We have a great deal of information about prevention of disease and disability in old age which is not being acted upon either by local authorities or by old people themselves. There are many popular misconceptions about old people, and one of the most widely held is that illness is synonymous with old age. In fact, many of us are fully active and independent, and our numbers should increase if we switch to a healthier diet and lifestyle. Here, too, orthodox curative medicine has made major contributions in such fields as hip replacement and cardiac surgery, has given many old people a new lease of life, and restored their autonomy and independence.

In our region of Italy, we estimate that nearly a quarter of the population will be over sixty-five by the year 2000, and the proportion of voters over sixty-five will obviously be even greater. This opens up the obvious opportunity to create an effective lobby for more adequate pensions, housing and community services for old people. What government, local authority or political party could possibly afford to ignore the demands of over a quarter of their voters? The pensioners' trade unions and some of the voluntary organizations are well aware of this, but relatively few old people seem to be actively involved.

In the book *Aspects of Aging* by Bernice Martin suggests that we are in the midst of a major revision of society's attitude toward old age at the present time. There is a growing number of four generation families, but in Britain, relatively few are in old people's homes, and the majority live independently. Since the Industrial Revolution, old age is synonymous with poverty for manual workers.

In Britain in the 1980's, 70 percent of the retired population relied on their state pension — the lowest in the Common Market — for their only source of income. Poverty and the illusion of powerlessness have been the hallmarks of old age for most workers.

We do not know how long we can live if we adopt a healthy diet and lifestyle. As far as I know, no one has yet organized a long-term trial of longevity in macrobiotics, and apart from Michio and Aveline Kushi, most of the followers of macrobiotics we have met have carried out the diet and lifestyle for less than twenty years, and have not yet entered the ranks of the third age. There have recently been forecasts in the press of life spans of 110, 120 and even 130 years, but these seem to have met with little general credence among scientists.

Susan Sontag has described the ways in which women are penalized in old age. It is much more important for a woman to feel desirable and preserve her physical appearance than for a man to. Aging tends to unsex women, whereas men can claim to be attractive for longer, especially if they possess the added advantages of money or power. The popularity of beauty care for those women who can afford it, and the fact that more men than women remarry after divorce, testify to this sex difference. Moreover, women live longer than men and they are still expected to care for aged relatives — often at a time when their own children have grown up and they could reasonably expect some leisure time for themselves.

There are dangers in this frantic search for eternal youth. Clearly few women are going to be able to compete with retired film stars, and even with the help of macrobiotics we are not all likely to enjoy a second adolescence. If we fail to make it, we may be accused of not trying hard enough. It's the old game of "blaming the victim." Of course, some people have managed to retain their beauty, energy and creativity well into the third age. But these are as exceptional as the young people who win open tennis tournaments and swimming championships in their early teens.

The attitude of society to old age has changed fundamentally, certainly in the United States and Western Europe. The image of old people as passive, helpless, unimportant, uninteresting and dreary, is fading fast. There are many reasons for this, and here I can only touch on one or two. Some ninety percent of all non-manual workers in the United States are now said to enjoy the benefits of occupational or private pension insurance schemes. Marketing firms have not failed to recognize a potential new market here, and the travel firm Argosy, which specializes in providing holidays for the older age group, is apparently highly successful. Evelina Curry, a previous junior Minister of Health, with a knack for the infelicitous phrase, speaks of the "Woopy," the well-off old person.

In the cinema, television and even detective stories, old people emerge as powerful personalities and, in the case of Monty Python's "Hell's Grannies," even violent. In Agatha Christie's novels, Miss Marple solves murders seated in her cottage in a peaceful English village, Compo and his mates pull off all the tricks in "The Last of the Summer Wine," Clive Dunn in "Dad's Army" frequently gets the better of his commanding officer. Figures of fun, yes, but far removed from the old biddies of the seaside postcards and Shakespeare's slippered pantaloon, shuffling to the grave.

Those of us already old are faced with a choice. We can either settle for a passive role, beset by fears of loss of status, loss of memory, vision, hearing or incapacitating disability and, for most of us, fear of poverty; or we can decide to take the initiative — to be bold. So where can we be bold? First, the enjoyment of leisure and retirement demands adequate financing. Today, in most Western countries there are many old people below the poverty line. This is clearly unacceptable. By leaving paid employment, we have not left society, which is still responsible for us.

At one of our Chianti workshops for old people, one participant said that the key question for him was freedom to choose, and that this implied an adequate income. We have to be able to decide whether we want to go on working, either full or part-time, where work exists. We must be free to choose whether to enter contributory state or private pension schemes. Here we need objective, accurate information and advice, and the pensioners' trade unions and voluntary bodies will have to provide experts in this complex field, and fully inform themselves.

We need a powerful lobby at the national and EEC level, where many of the decisions affecting old people will be made in coming years. We need to lobby all political parties, and play an active role in the pensioners' trade unions and old people's organizations. We have to emerge from our isolation and helplessness and discover our potential strength.

At local authority level much remains to be done. There are enormous differences in the provisions for old people's housing, health and social services, and leisure facilities both in the countries we know best and in different areas within each country. It is too soon to say whether the new provisions in general practice in Britain will help or hinder the health care of old people. A great deal is known about preventive measures in the community in old age and we have to insist that all local authority services rise to the level of the best. Space does not allow us to go into details on this subject here, but we are preparing a book which will inform our fellow senior citizens on what they can do, and supply them with ammunition for the battles ahead.

How can we ourselves be bold? First, we can respond to the opportunities presented by the present climate of opinion. Everywhere authoritarianism is being rejected, men and women are demanding liberty, and the old can break their chains. We are all individuals with the capacity to change and grow at almost any age. We all have enormous resources, for the most part unused. Old age can become a time for adventure when we cheerfully go out to meet new challenges. To be able to do this we need to be as fit as possible. We need to look at our diet and our way of life. We believe a macrobiotic diet can make us healthier in old age, can improve the quality of our lives and perhaps help us to live longer. But even if we are not all prepared to embark on the macrobiotic path, there is plenty of evidence from orthodox dietitians that old people do better on less animal fat, less refined salt and sugar, few if any cigarettes, little alcohol, and with more grains and vegetables. When we retire, we tend to sit around more, when in fact we need regular exercise to keep fit. This can take the form we prefer — walking, swimming, tennis, bowling, keep-fit exercises — whatever we prefer. The important thing is to enjoy whatever we choose and not to try to break any records!

Lastly, all kinds of activity are good. Old age is a time for doing the things you've always wanted to do. You will be surprised how much energy you have. If you missed out on study and education the first time round, what about the University of the Third Age, local authority hobby and language classes, music and acting? Never were there so many opportunities. We can make sure our minority interests are catered to. Never was there a better time for old people to be bold! It's up to us to see that we have the right to spend our old age in the way we choose.

1. Jefferys, M. *Aspects of Aging.*

Afterword

"A fountain breaks out in the wilderness, but that fountain cares not whether any man comes to fetch water or no; a fresh and fit gale blows upon the sea, but it cares not whether the mariners hoist sail or no; a rose blows in your garden, but it calls you not to smell it."

— John Donne

Hugh: I am convinced that a macrobiotic diet and life style can make most of us healthier and help to prevent many diseases. It may well prolong life, and if it does not add "years to life" it can certainly add "life to your years." We need properly conducted clinical trials on the effect of a macrobiotic regime on various types of established chronic illness, and long term trials of its role in prevention and health promotion. The unfortunate experience of the Bristol Center teaches us that such research must be very carefully planned at every stage. The anecdotal evidence we have provided won't convince many of my medical colleagues.

From my own personal experience it is clear that in cases where orthodox medicine can offer no effective treatment, a percentage of patients can recover. I firmly believe that we can directly influence this result by adopting a macrobiotic way of life — a positive outlook, a healthy diet, physical and mental activity, fresh air, pure water, getting as close to nature as we can — and, about all, love and hope! If our book can help others to realize this objective it will have achieved its aim.

Marian: It is over five years since our adventure in the world of macrobiotics first began. How do I feel about it all now? Every morning I wake up and feel deeply grateful that Hugh is alive and so well. We share most things in life — reading, writing, housework, shopping, cooking, swimming, walking, gardening, and loving. We go to our office in the new library of the local authority three times a week. Here we are helping to organize research into the loss of autonomy in old people, and trying to set up an enquiry bureau for health — *amica salute,* or "health, your friend." This will tell the general public about the health and social services available and the various self-help and complementary health organizations.

Fortunately there is a sports club with a warm championship pool near our office and we swim there in the lunch hour. We also join a keep-fit class twice a week. We both feel better for the exercise and hope to do more walking in our spare time.

When Hugh got ill we thought all this would come to an end, yet within three months of his diagnosis in London we were back in Italy working happily again and with more plans than before! I feel as if we have shared Hugh's illness too — shared the shock, the fear, the pain and then the hope and happiness. Certainly we have grown closer together accepting the challenge of a new diet and way of life.

In macrobiotics we soon made new friends among the people we met at conferences, workshops and camps. I like the idea of consciously living closer to nature, of eating whole and pure foods, of seeking to recreate our natural balance. I have enjoyed telling Hugh's story, and hoping that it can convince others to help their bodies overcome cancer. I am certain that shiatsu can be of physical, mental, and spiritual benefit to most people. Hugh had weekly sessions during the first two years after diagnosis, and it helped him greatly. I used to go with him to watch and learn, and I noticed the improvement after each visit. Now he continues to go from time to time to our good friend Gioachino Allasia in Florence. We also sometimes give each other shiatsu at home.

Today our world is full of suffering. The earth, sea, and air are polluted from our ignorance and contempt for nature. I believe that a positive commitment to a healthy diet and lifestyle can begin to influence society and help to create a happy, peaceful, and healthy future for all living beings — One Peaceful World.

Appendix

Standard Macrobiotic Dietary Guidelines*

Foods for Daily Consumption

• **Whole Cereal Grains:** The principal food of each meal is daily whole cereal grain, comprising from 50 to 60 percent of the total volume. Whole grains include brown rice, whole wheat berries, barley, millet, and rye, as well as corn, buckwheat, and other botanically similar plants. From time to time, whole grain products, such as cracked wheat, rolled oats, noodles, pasta, bread, baked goods, and other unrefined flour products, may be served as part of this volume.

• **Soup:** One to two small bowls of soup, making up about 5 to 10 percent of daily food intake, are consumed each day. The soup broth is made frequently with miso or shoyu and also includes vegetable, bean, and grain soups.

• **Vegetables:** About 25 to 30 percent of daily food includes fresh vegetables prepared in a variety of ways, including steaming, boiling, baking, sautéing, salads, and marinades. The vegetables include a variety of root vegetables (such as cabbage, carrots, and daikon radish), ground vegetables (such as onions and fall-

and winter-season squashes), and leafy green vegetables (such as kale, collard greens, broccoli, turnip greens, mustard greens, and watercress).

• **Beans and Sea Vegetables:** A small portion, about 10 percent by volume, of daily food intake includes cooked beans such as adukis, lentils, and chickpeas or bean products such as tofu, tempeh, and natto and sea vegetables, including kombu, wakame, nori, dulse, hijiki, and arame.

• **Seasoning and Oil:** Naturally processed sea salt is used in seasoning, along with miso, shoyu, umeboshi, brown rice vinegar, fresh grated ginger and other traditional items. Naturally processed, unrefined vegetable oil is recommended for daily cooking such as dark sesame seed oil. Kuzu is commonly used for gravies and sauces.

• **Condiments:** Condiments include gomashio (roasted sesame salt), roasted seaweed powders, umeboshi plums, tekka root vegetables, and many others.

• **Pickles:** A small volume of home-made pickles is eaten each day to aid in digestion of grains and vegetables.

• **Beverages:** Spring or well water is used for drinking, preparing tea, and for general cooking. Bancha twig tea (also known as kukicha) is the most commonly served beverage, though roasted barley tea, and other grain-based teas or traditional, non-stimulant herbal teas are also used frequently.

Occasional Foods for Those in Usual Good Health

• **Animal Food:** A small volume of white-meat fish or seafood may be eaten a few times per week.

• **Seeds and Nuts:** Seeds and nuts, lightly roasted and salted with sea salt or seasoned with shoyu, may be enjoyed as occasional snacks.

• **Fruit:** Fruit may be taken a few times a week, preferably cooked or naturally dried, as a snack or dessert, provided the fruit grows in the local or similar climate zone.

• **Dessert:** Occasional desserts may consist of cookies, pudding, cake, pie, and other dishes made with naturally sweet foods such as apples, fall- and winter-season squashes, aduki beans, or dried fruit or may be sweetened with a natural grain-based sweetener such as amasake, barley malt, or rice syrup.

* *These guidelines are for four-season temperate climates including most of the United States and Canada, Europe, Russia, and China. For guidelines for tropical, semitropical, polar, and semipolar climates, please see Michio Kushi,* Standard Macrobiotic Diet *(One Peaceful World Press, 1991).*

Way of Life Suggestions

• Live each day happily without being preoccupied with your health; try to keep mentally and physically active.

• View everything and everyone you meet with gratitude, particularly offering thanks before and after every meal.

• Please chew your food very well, at least 50 times per mouthful, or until it becomes liquid.

• It is best to avoid wearing synthetic or woolen clothes directly on the skin. As much as possible, wear cotton, especially for undergarments. Avoid excessive metallic accessories on the fingers, wrists, or neck. Keep such ornaments simple and graceful.

• If your strength permits, go outdoors in simple clothing. Walk on the grass, beach, or soil up to one-half hour every day. Keep your home in good order, from the kitchen, bathroom, bedroom, and living rooms, to every corner of the house.

• Initiate and maintain an active correspondence, extending your best wishes to parents, children, brothers and sisters, teachers, and friends.

• Avoid taking long hot baths or showers unless you have been consuming too much salt or animal food.

• To increase circulation, scrub your entire body with a hot, damp towel every morning or every night. If that is not possible, at least scrub your hands, feet, fingers, and toes.

• Avoid chemically perfumed cosmetics. For care of the

teeth, brush with natural preparations or sea salt.

• If your condition permits, exercise regularly as part of daily life, including activities like walking, scrubbing floors, cleaning windows, washing clothes and working in the garden. You may also participate in exercise programs such as yoga, martial arts, dance, or sports.

• Avoid using electric cooing devices (ovens and ranges) or microwave ovens. Convert to gas or wood-stove cooking at the earliest opportunity.

• It is best to minimize the use of color television and computer display units.

• Include some large green plants in your house to freshen and enrich the oxygen content of the air of your home.

• Sing a happy song each day.

These guidelines are intended to supplement consultation with a medical or nutritional professional or personal guidance received from a qualified macrobiotic teacher.

The publishers wish to express our gratitude and support to the following organizations for their dietary recommendations as expressed in their publications:

Dietary Goals for the United States, published in 1977 (revised in 1980) by the U.S. Senate Select Committee on Nutrition and Human Needs.

Healthy People: Health Promotion and Disease Prevention, published in 1979 by the U.S. Surgeon General.

Diet, Nutrition, and Cancer, published in 1982 by the National Academy of Sciences.

Diet and Health, published in 1989 by the National Academy of Sciences.

The China Health Study, published in 1990 by the U.S. National Cancer Institute and the Chinese Institute of Nutrition and Food Hygiene.

The New Four Food Groups, published in 1991 by the Physicians Committee for Responsible Medicine.

Diet, Nutrition, and the Prevention of Chronic Diseases, published in 1991 by the World Health Organization Study Group on Diet, Nutrition, and Prevention of Noncommunicable Diseases.

Reports, statements, and dietary guidelines made by the:

- American Heart Assocation
- American Diabetes Association
- American Society for Clinical Nutrition
- American Cancer Society

Resources

One Peaceful World

One Peaceful World is an international information network and friendship society founded by Michio and Aveline Kushi. Its members include individuals, familes, educational centers, organic farmers, teachers, parents and children, authors and artists, homemakers and business people, and others devoted to the realization of one healthy, peaceful world. Activities include educational and spiritual tours, assemblies and forums, international food aid and environmental awareness, One Peaceful World Press, and other activities to help humanity pass safely into a new world of planetary health and peace.

Annual membership is $30 for individuals, $50 for families, and $100 for supporting members. Benefits include the quarterly *One Peaceful World Newsletter*, discounts of selected books, cassettes, and videos, and special mailings and communications.

To enroll or for further information, contact:

One Peaceful World
Box 10
Becket, MA 01223
(413) 623-2322
Fax (413) 623-8827

Kushi Institute — Michio Kushi Seminars

Studies in Destiny—In these ongoing seminars presented at the Kushi Institute of the Berkshires, Michio Kushi presents fascinating and revealing studies of the way to see, judge, and freely manage both personal destiny and planetary destiny based on yin and yang, the art of physiognomy and the art of environmental placement and household arrangement.

Spiritual Training Seminars—These ongoing seminars presented at the Kushi Institute of the Berkshires, are part of a progressive series designed to enhance each person's capacity for self-realization and fulfillment.

New Medicine for Humanity—In this series of seminars, Michio Kushi offers ongoing studies on the origin and development of health, the relation of diet and degenerative disease, and the reorientation of modern society in a healthier, more peaceful direction.

All seminars include macrobiotic/vegetarian meals. For dates, costs, and to register, or for more information, contact:

Kushi Institute of the Berkshires
Box 7
Becket, MA 01223
(413) 623-5741
Fax (413) 623-8827

Recommended Reading

Books

1. *AIDS, Macrobiotics, and Natural Immunity.* Michio Kushi, with Martha Cotrell, M.D. Japan Publications, 1990, paperback, $19.95.

2. *Amber Waves of Grain.* Alex and Gale Jack, Japan Publications, 1992, paperback, $17.00.

3. *Basic Home Remedies.* Michio Kushi. One Peaceful World Press, 1994, paperback, $6.95.

4. *The Book of Do In.* Michio Kushi. Japan Publications, 1979, paperback, $14.95.

5. *The Book of Macrobiotics.* Michio Kushi with Alex Jack. Japan Publications, 1986, paperback, $15.95.

6. *Cancer-Free: 30 Who Triumphed Over Cancer Naturally.* East West Foundation, with Ann Fawcett and Cynthia Smith. Japan Publications, 1992, paperback, $15.95.

7. *The Cancer-Prevention Diet.* Michio Kushi with Alex Jack. St. Martin's Press, 1993; hardcover, $24.95.

8. *Diet for a Strong Heart.* Michio Kushi with Alex Jack. St. Martin's Press, 1985, paperback, $10.95.

9. *Food Governs Your Destiny.* Michio and Aveline Kushi, with Alex Jack. Japan Publications, 1991, paperback, $12.95.

10. *Healing Harvest.* Michio Kushi with Edward Esko. One Peaceful World Press, 1994, paperback, $9.95.

11. *Healing Planet Earth.* Edward Esko. One Peaceful World Press, 1992, paperback, $5.95.

12. *Holistic Health Through Macrobiotics.* Michio Kushi with Edward Esko. Japan Publications, 1994, paperback, $18.00.

13. *How to See Your Health.* Michio Kushi. Japan Publications, 1980, paperback, $12.95.

14. *Inspector Ginkgo Tips His Hat to Sherlock Holmes.* Alex Jack. One Peaceful World Press, 1994, paperback, $12.95.

15. *Let Food Be Thy Medicine.* Alex Jack. One Peaceful World Press, updated and revised, 1994, paperback, $10.95.

16. *The Macrobiotic Approach to Cancer.* Michio Kushi, with Edward Esko. Avery Publishing Group, 1991, paperback, $9.95.

17. *Macrobiotic Diet.* Micho and Aveline Kushi, with Alex Jack. Japan Publications, 1993, paperback, $17.00.

18. *Macrobiotic Home Food Processing.* Guy Lalumiere, One Peaceful World Press, 1993, paperback, $8.95.

19. *Macrobiotic Palm Healing.* Michio Kushi, with Olivia Oredson. Japan Publications, 1989, paperback, $15.95.

20. *Macrobiotics and Oriental Medicine.* Michio Kushi with Phillip Jannetta. Japan Publications, 1991, paperback, $18.95.

21. *Natural Healing through Macrobiotics.* Michio Kushi, with Edward Esko and Marc Van Cauwenberghe, M.D. Japan Publications, 1979, paperback, $14.95.

22. *Nine Star Ki.* Michio Kushi, with Edward Esko. One Peaceful World Press, 1991, paperback, $12.95.

23. *Notes from the Boundless Frontier.* Edward Esko. One Peaceful World Press, 1992, paperback, $5.95.

24. *One Peaceful World.* Michio Kushi with Alex Jack. St. Martin's Press, 1987, hardcover, $17.95.

25. *Other Dimensions: Exploring the Unexplained.* Michio Kushi with Edward Esko. Avery Publishing Group, 1991, paperback, $9.95.

26. *Out of Thin Air: A Comedy About Owls and Ozone, Beef and Biodiversity, Grains and Global Warming.* Alex Jack. One Peaceful World Press, 1993, paperback, $7.95.

27. *The Philosopher's Stone.* Michio Kushi with Edward Esko. One Peaceful World Press, 1994, paperback, $9.95.

28. *Physician Heal Thyself.* Dr. Hugh Faulkner. One Peaceful World Press, 1992, paperback, $7.95.

29. *Promenade Home: Macrobiotics and Women's Health.* Gale and Alex Jack. Japan Publications,1988, paperback, $18.95.

30. *The Pulse of Life.* Edward Esko. One Peaceful World Press, 1994, paperback, $7.95.

31. *Recovery: From Cancer to Health through Macrobiotics.* Elaine Nussbaum. Avery Publishing Group, 1993, paperback, $9.95

32. *Standard Macrobiotic Diet.* Michio Kushi. One Peaceful World Press, 1991, paperback, $5.95.

33. *Your Face Never Lies.* Michio Kushi. Avery Publishing Group, 1983, paperback, $9.95.

Publications

One Peaceful World, Becket, Massachusetts
MacroNews, Philadelphia, Pennsylvania
Macrobiotics Today, Oroville, California

Books by Mail Order

The books listed above are available by mail-order from One Peaceful World Press. Please make check or money order payable to One Peaceful World and enclose shipping and handling of $2.00 for the first book and $1.00 for each additional book.

Outside U.S., please pay in U.S. funds drawn on a U.S. bank and enclose 20% of total order for surface mail and 40% for airmail.

Visa or Mastercard also accepted in payment. Please enclose card number, expiration date, and authorized signature.

Note: Prices subject to change.

About the Authors

Dr. Hugh Faulkner served as a General Practitioner in his native Britain for many years. His wife, Marian, is a nurse. They are now living near Florence, Italy, and are active in a variety of educational and publishing projects.

Join One Peaceful World, the Global Macrobiotic Information Network & Friendship Society

Join One Peaceful World, the association of macrobiotic friends and families around the world, and become part of a planetary network devoted to creating a healthy, peaceful world.

Benefits include:

- A Membership Card
- A subscription to the quarterly One Peaceful World Newsletter with macrobiotic news from around the world, medical-scientific updates, cancer case history reports, articles by Michio Kushi, recipes, book and movie reviews, etc.
- A free book from One Peaceful World Press
- 10% discount of new books and selected study materials

Individual membership is $30.00/year
Family membership is $50.00/year
Supporting membership is $100.00/year

Send name and address and check payable to One Peaceful World to Box 10, Becket MA 01223. Visa/MC also accepted.